T0229220

Dentoalveolar Surgery

Editor

MICHAEL A. KLEIMAN

ORAL AND MAXILLOFACIAL SURGERY CLINICS OF NORTH AMERICA

www.oralmaxsurgery.theclinics.com

Consulting Editor
RICHARD H. HAUG

August 2015 • Volume 27 • Number 3

ELSEVIER

1600 John F. Kennedy Boulevard • Suite 1800 • Philadelphia, Pennsylvania, 19103-2899

http://www.oralmaxsurgery.theclinics.com

ORAL AND MAXILLOFACIAL SURGERY CLINICS OF NORTH AMERICA Volume 27, Number 3
August 2015 ISSN 1042-3699, ISBN-13: 978-0-323-39348-5

Editor: John Vassallo; j.vassallo@elsevier.com
Developmental Editor: Colleen Viola

© 2015 Elsevier Inc. All rights reserved.

This periodical and the individual contributions contained in it are protected under copyright by Elsevier, and the following terms and conditions apply to their use:

Photocopying

Single photocopies of single articles may be made for personal use as allowed by national copyright laws. Permission of the Publisher and payment of a fee is required for all other photocopying, including multiple or systematic copying, copying for advertising or promotional purposes, resale, and all forms of document delivery. Special rates are available for educational institutions that wish to make photocopies for non-profit educational classroom use. For information on how to seek permission visit www.elsevier.com/permissions or call: (+44) 1865 843830 (UK)/(+1) 215 239 3804 (USA).

Derivative Works

Subscribers may reproduce tables of contents or prepare lists of articles including abstracts for internal circulation within their institutions. Permission of the Publisher is required for resale or distribution outside the institution. Permission of the Publisher is required for all other derivative works, including compilations and translations (please consult www.elsevier.com/permissions).

Electronic Storage or Usage

Permission of the Publisher is required to store or use electronically any material contained in this periodical, including any article or part of an article (please consult www.elsevier.com/permissions). Except as outlined above, no part of this publication may be reproduced, stored in a retrieval system or transmitted in any form or by any means, electronic, mechanical, photocopying, recording or otherwise, without prior written permission of the Publisher.

Notice

No responsibility is assumed by the Publisher for any injury and/or damage to persons or property as a matter of products liability, negligence or otherwise, or from any use or operation of any methods, products, instructions or ideas contained in the material herein. Because of rapid advances in the medical sciences, in particular, independent verification of diagnoses and drug dosages should be made.

Although all advertising material is expected to conform to ethical (medical) standards, inclusion in this publication does not constitute a guarantee or endorsement of the quality or value of such product or of the claims made of it by its manufacturer.

Oral and Maxillofacial Surgery Clinics of North America (ISSN 1042-3699) is published quarterly by Elsevier Inc., 360 Park Avenue South, New York, NY 10010-1710. Months of issue are February, May, August, and November. Business and Editorial Offices: 1600 John F. Kennedy Blvd., Suite 1800, Philadelphia, PA 19103-2899. Periodicals postage paid at New York, NY and additional mailing offices. Subscription prices are $385.00 per year for US individuals, $567.00 per year for US institutions, $175.00 per year for US students and residents, $455.00 per year for Canadian individuals, $680.00 per year for Canadian institutions, $520.00 per year for international individuals, $680.00 per year for international institutions and $235.00 per year for Canadian and foreign students/residents. To receive student/resident rate, orders must be accompanied by name or affiliated institution, date of term, and the *signature* of program/residency coordinator on institution letterhead. Orders will be billed at individual rate until proof of status is received. Foreign air speed delivery is included in all *Clinics* subscription prices. All prices are subject to change without notice. **POSTMASTER:** Send address changes to *Oral and Maxillofacial Surgery Clinics of North America,* Elsevier Periodicals **Customer Service, 11830 Westline Industrial Drive, St. Louis, MO 63146. Tel: 1-800-654-2452 (U.S. and Canada); 314-447-8871 (outside U.S. and Canada). Fax: 314-447-8029. E-mail: journals customerservice-usa@elsevier.com (for print support); journalsonlinesupport-usa@elsevier.com (for online support).**

Reprints. For copies of 100 or more, of articles in this publication, please contact the Commercial Reprints Department, Elsevier Inc., 360 Park Avenue South, New York, NY 10010-1710. Tel.: 212-633-3874; Fax: 212-633-3820; Email: reprints@elsevier.com.

Oral and Maxillofacial Surgery Clinics of North America is covered in *MEDLINE/PubMed (Index Medicus), Science Citation Index Expanded (SciSearch®), Journal Citation Reports/Science Edition,* and *Current Contents®/Clinical Medicine.*

Contributors

CONSULTING EDITOR

RICHARD H. HAUG, DDS
Professor and Chief, Oral Maxillofacial Surgery,
Carolinas Medical Center, Charlotte, North
Carolina

EDITOR

MICHAEL A. KLEIMAN, DMD
Private Practice, Oral and Maxillofacial
Surgery, Edison-Clark Oral Surgery
Associates, Edison, New Jersey

AUTHORS

SHELLY ABRAMOWICZ, DMD, MPH
Assistant Professor, Division of Oral and
Maxillofacial Surgery, Department of Surgery,
Emory University School of Medicine, Atlanta,
Georgia

ADRIAN BECKER, BDS, LDS, DDO
Clinical Associate Professor Emeritus,
Department of Orthodontics, Hebrew
University-Hadassah School of Dental
Medicine, Jerusalem, Israel

MICHAEL S. BLOCK, DMD
Private Practice, Metairie, Louisiana

STELLA CHAUSHU, DMD, MSc, PhD
Associate Professor and Chair, Department
of Orthodontics, Hebrew University-Hadassah
School of Dental Medicine, Jerusalem,
Israel

GEORGE R. DEEB, DDS, MD
Associate Professor, Department of Oral and
Maxillofacial Surgery, School of Dentistry,
Virginia Commonwealth University, Richmond,
Virginia

JANINA GOLOB DEEB, DDS, MS
Assistant Professor, Departments of
Periodontics and General Practice, School of

Dentistry, Virginia Commonwealth University,
Richmond, Virginia

STEPHANIE J. DREW, DMD
Assistant Clinical Professor, Hofstra Medical
School, Hofstra University, Hempstead, New
York; Assistant Clinical Professor, University
Hospital Stony Brook, Stony Brook,
New York; The New York Center for
Orthognathic and Maxillofacial Surgery, West
Islip, New York

HILLEL EPHROS, DMD, MD
Program Director, Oral and Maxillofacial
Surgery; Chairman, Department of Dentistry,
Medical Director of the Regional Craniofacial
Center, St. Joseph's Regional Medical Center,
Paterson, New Jersey

JAMES R. HUPP, DMD, MD, JD, MBA
Founding Dean and Professor of Oral-
Maxillofacial Surgery, School of Dental
Medicine, East Carolina University, Greenville,
North Carolina

ROBERT KLEIN, DDS
Chief Resident, Oral and Maxillofacial Surgery,
St. Joseph's Regional Medical Center,
Paterson, New Jersey

STUART E. LIEBLICH, DMD
Clinical Professor, Oral and Maxillofacial
Surgery, University of Connecticut Health
Center, Farmington, Connecticut; Private
Practice, Avon Oral and Maxillofacial Surgery,
Avon, Connecticut

SAMI A. NIZAM II, DMD, MD
Resident, Department of Oral and Maxillofacial
Surgery, Rutgers University School of Dental
Medicine, Newark, New Jersey

**M. ANTHONY POGREL, DDS, MD, FRCS,
FACS**
Professor of Oral and Maxillofacial Surgery,
Department of Oral and Maxillofacial Surgery,
University of California San Francisco, San
Francisco, California

LOUIS K. RAFETTO, DMD
Director of Surgical Implantology and Alveolar
Reconstruction, Department of Oral and

Maxillofacial Surgery and Hospital Dentistry,
Christiana Care Health System, Wilmington,
Delaware

STEVEN M. ROSER, DMD, MD
DeLos Hill Professor of Oral Surgery;
Chief, Division of Oral and Maxillofacial
Surgery, Department of Surgery, Emory
University School of Medicine, Atlanta,
Georgia

ANTHONY SALLUSTIO, DDS
Chief, Prosthodontics and Maxillofacial
Prosthetics, St. Joseph's Regional Medical
Center, Paterson, New Jersey

VINCENT B. ZICCARDI, DDS, MD, FACS
Professor, Chair and Residency Director,
Department of Oral and Maxillofacial Surgery,
Rutgers University School of Dental Medicine,
Newark, New Jersey

Contents

Medical Management of Patients Undergoing Dentoalveolar Surgery 345

Shelly Abramowicz and Steven M. Roser

> The oral and maxillofacial surgeon (OMS) should have an understanding of common medical comorbidities. This understanding allows for risk stratification and thus prevention of potential problems. Remaining knowledgeable regarding diseases, diagnosis, treatment strategies, and pharmacology ultimately improves patient care. This article provides an update on some of the most common medical diseases for the patient undergoing dentoalveolar surgery.

Dental Extractions and Preservation of Space for Implant Placement in Molar Sites 353

Michael S. Block

> The clinician is often asked to remove a tooth and place an implant into the site. The implant must be placed with appropriate stability to allow for integration to occur, which requires bone presence. Bone is also necessary to allow for ideal implant positioning within the alveolus for functional and esthetic concerns. The purpose of this article is to discuss the changes in socket dimensions over time and how to promote space maintenance, with an algorithm for treatment based on evidence.

Managing Impacted Third Molars 363

Louis K. Rafetto

> Oral and maxillofacial surgeons can be reasonably certain of the behavior of wisdom teeth and the outcomes of different management strategies. An organized approach based on symptom and disease status simplifies management recommendations. The patients who provide the greatest challenge to certainty are those whose wisdom teeth are asymptomatic and disease free. Patients who elect to retain a third molar should be advised about this risk of removal over time. Given the increased complication rate when third molars are removed with increasing age, it may be prudent to extract them by the middle of the third decade.

Coronectomy: Partial Odontectomy or Intentional Root Retention 373

M. Anthony Pogrel

> Coronectomy is considered in patients older than 25, where there is an intimate relationship between the roots of a retained lower third molar (occasionally second or first molars) and the inferior alveolar nerve, in noncontraindicated circumstances. It may be used on younger patients with a medium to high risk of inferior alveolar nerve damage. The decision to use this technique is made with the aid of cone-beam computed tomography scans. Short- to medium-term success rate is excellent, but long-term studies are not yet available. The technique is gaining wider acceptance, although there are differences in the indications and actual technique used within and between countries.

teeth and implants. These tools should be in the armamentarium of oral and maxillofacial surgeons providing implant services.

ORAL AND MAXILLOFACIAL SURGERY CLINICS OF NORTH AMERICA

RELATED INTEREST

Dental Clinics of North America July 2015 (Vol. 59, No. 3)
Modern Concepts in Aesthetic Dentistry and Multi-disciplined Reconstructive Grand Rounds
John R. Calamia, Richard D. Trushkowsky, Steven B. David, and Mark S. Wolff, *Editors*
Available at: www.dental.theclinics.com

THE CLINICS ARE NOW AVAILABLE ONLINE!
Access your subscription at:
www.theclinics.com

Preface
Achieving and Maintaining Excellence in Dentoalveolar Surgery

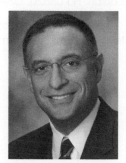

Michael A. Kleiman, DMD
Editor

Oral and maxillofacial surgery (OMS) is a specialty that has significantly expanded in scope far beyond the limits of the oral cavity. However, dentoalveolar surgery is where it began as a specialty and where it began for many individuals as practitioners. As a general topic, dentoalveolar surgery is not the most glamorous or impressive of the things we do. In fact, it may not even be listed by some of our surgical residents when they are asked to explain what the specialty of OMS is. Despite that, it is the thing that most oral and maxillofacial surgeons do the most of and what many, if not most of us, have a passion for.

Jim Collins, in his book *Good to Great*, teaches that an organization should determine where to direct its energy by examining the intersection of three circles. They are:

1. What you have a passion for
2. What drives your economic engine
3. What you can be the best in the world at

Clearly, for the specialty of Oral and Maxillofacial Surgery, the area of dentoalveolar surgery falls solidly within the intersection of these three circles.

As basic as it is in some respects, dentoalveolar surgery has evolved and changed significantly. The advent of modern dental implants and readily available 3-dimensional imaging techniques have altered our objectives and changed the ways that we sometimes measure "excellence." In addition, we have seen other specialties expand their scopes. They are trying to become expert in areas that were once solely the province of the specialty of Oral and Maxillofacial Surgery.

To keep dentoalveolar surgery within the intersection of our specialty's "three circles," we as practitioners must be sure to continue to be the "best in the world" at what we do. The "mission" of this issue of *Oral and Maxillofacial Surgery Clinics of North America* is to help us as oral and maxillofacial surgeons achieve and maintain that goal. We as oral and maxillofacial surgeons cannot take our ability in dentoalveolar surgery for granted. It must be approached in the same way as all of the other "sexy" things that we do!

At the outset, I tried not to cross the line into other topics that may be covered in other issues of *Oral and Maxillofacial Surgery Clinics of North America*. However, it soon became clear that this is not possible or appropriate. One cannot talk about extraction techniques, hard and soft tissue grafting, or preprosthetic surgery without also considering the world of dental implants. Nor can one expose an impacted canine with a high level of "excellence" without appreciating what the orthodontist's perspective is in the treatment of the patient. As an overall umbrella, we must operate within a "Culture of Safety," to protect our patients, coworkers, and ourselves.

I greatly appreciate the tremendous contributions of each and every one of our authors. I am sure that any oral and maxillofacial surgeon looking at the table of contents will be struck

Oral Maxillofacial Surg Clin N Am 27 (2015) ix–x
http://dx.doi.org/10.1016/j.coms.2015.05.001
1042-3699/15/$ – see front matter © 2015 Published by Elsevier Inc.

by the collection of experts and leaders in their fields who have worked hard to contribute to this effort. I am grateful to Dr. Richard Haug for asking me to edit this issue and recognizing the importance of the topic. I would also like to recognize the excellence of the publishing staff at Elsevier.

Last, I must recognize and thank my wife, Frayda, for convincing me to take on this project. I initially told Rich Haug that I didn't think I would have the time to take on this additional work, but she said, "You have to do this!" She was right, and I guess I did!

Michael A. Kleiman, DMD
Oral and Maxillofacial Surgery
Edison-Clark Oral Surgery Associates
1857 Oak Tree Road
Edison, NJ 08820, USA

E-mail address:
kleiman710@gmail.com

Medical Management of Patients Undergoing Dentoalveolar Surgery

Shelly Abramowicz, DMD, MPH*, Steven M. Roser, DMD, MD

KEYWORDS

- Medical management • Dentoalveolar surgery • Anticoagulation
- Medication-related osteonecrosis

KEY POINTS

- Presurgical evaluation should include risk stratification for prevention of potential problems.
- There are new guidelines regarding management of patients taking oral anticoagulants.
- There is a recent update regarding management of patients with medication-related osteonecrosis of the jaw (MRONJ).

INTRODUCTION

The oral and maxillofacial surgeon (OMS) should have an understanding of common medical co-morbidities. This understanding allows for risk stratification and thus prevention of potential problems. Remaining current with updated literature regarding diseases, diagnosis, treatment strategies, and pharmacology ultimately improves patient care. This article provides an update on some of the most common medical diseases for the patient undergoing dentoalveolar surgery.

PRESURGICAL EVALUATION

Preoperative evaluation begins with a complete history and physical examination. First, the patient completes a screening questionnaire, which includes medical and surgical histories, allergies, and a list of current medications. The patient is then classified according to the American Society of Anesthesiologists (ASA) Physical Status Classification System (**Table 1**). The ASA classification system provides an overall impression of a surgical patient who is to undergo a procedure under anesthesia. The patient's risk of having a complication is then stratified according to the Surgical Classification System (**Table 2**).

CARDIOVASCULAR

When meeting a patient, the OMS should begin with a cardiac-focused physical examination. This examination consists of obtaining blood pressure in both arms, assessing for carotid/jugular pulsations/bruits/murmurs, examining the abdomen for distension and hepatosplenomegaly, and assessing the extremities for peripheral edema. One or more of these findings may alert the surgeon that decompensated cardiac disease is present. Next, the surgeon should consider clinical predictors of increased perioperative cardiovascular risk. The American Heart Association and American College of Cardiology determined that a patient who has specific cardiac clinical risks should be further evaluated by a cardiologist for additional cardiac risk stratification (**Table 3**). Next, the OMS should evaluate the patient's functional status using activities of daily living and

Division of Oral and Maxillofacial Surgery, Department of Surgery, Emory University, School of Medicine, 1365 Clifton Road, Northeast, Building B, Suite 2300, Atlanta, GA, USA
* Corresponding author. Division of Oral and Maxillofacial Surgery, Department of Surgery, Emory University, School of Medicine, 1365 Clifton Road, Northeast, Building B, Suite 2300, Atlanta, GA 30306.
E-mail address: sabram5@emory.edu

Oral Maxillofacial Surg Clin N Am 27 (2015) 345–352
http://dx.doi.org/10.1016/j.coms.2015.04.005
1042-3699/15/$ – see front matter © 2015 Elsevier Inc. All rights reserved.

Table 1
American Society of Anesthesiologists patient classification

ASA PS	Preoperative Health Status	Comments and Examples
1	Normal healthy patient	No organic, physiologic, or psychiatric disturbance; healthy with good exercise tolerance
2	Mild systemic disease	No functional limitations; has a well-controlled disease of 1 body system Examples: controlled hypertension without systemic effects, cigarette smoking without COPD, mild obesity, pregnancy
3	Severe systemic disease	Some functional limitation; has a controlled disease of more than 1 body system or 1 major system with no immediate danger of death Examples: controlled CHF, stable angina, poorly controlled hypertension, morbid obesity, chronic renal failure
4	Severe systemic disease that is a constant threat to life	Has at least 1 severe disease that is poorly controlled or at end stage; possible risk of death Examples: unstable angina, symptomatic COPD, symptomatic CHF, hepatorenal failure
5	Moribund, not expected to survive without the operation	Not expected to survive more than 24 h without surgery; imminent risk of death Examples: multiorgan failure, sepsis syndrome with hemodynamic instability, poorly controlled coagulopathy
6	Declared brain dead, organ donor	—

Note: if a surgical procedure is performed emergently, "E" is added to the previously defined ASA classification.
Abbreviations: CHF, congestive heart failure; COPD, chronic obstructive pulmonary disease.
Adapted from ASA Physical Status Classification System. American Society of Anesthesiologists. Available at: https://www.asahq.org/resources/clinical-information/asa-physical-status-classification-system; with permission.

Table 2
Surgical classification system

Category 1	Minimal risk to patients independent of anesthesia Minimally invasive procedures with little or no blood loss Operation done in an office setting
Category 2	Minimal to moderately invasive procedures Blood loss<500 mL Mild risk to patients independent of anesthesia
Category 3	Moderately to significantly invasive procedure Blood loss 500–1000 mL Moderate risk to patients independent of anesthesia
Category 4	Highly invasive procedure Blood loss>1500 mL Major risk to patients independent of anesthesia

From Fattahi T. Perioperative laboratory and diagnostic testing–what is needed and when? Oral Maxillofac Surg Clin North Am 2006;18(1):3, v; with permission.

metabolic equivalents (METs). One MET is the oxygen consumption of a 70-kg, 40-year-old at rest. A patient who is able to perform activities of greater than 4 METs without symptoms is considered to have a good functional capacity (**Table 4**).[1] Finally, the Goldman criteria relies on multivariate analysis and assigns points to certain physical characteristics, helping to assess a patient's cardiac risk (**Table 5**). The points are then tallied and correlated with the cardiac risk.[2] Patients range from having 0 points and thus a 0.9% risk of serious cardiac event or death to greater than 26 points and a 63.6% risk of serious cardiac event or death.[2]

Hypertension

Hypertension is defined as blood pressure higher than 140/90 mm Hg measured on 2 different occasions over a 1- to 2-week span. The Joint National Committee on Prevention, Detection, Evaluation, and Treatment of High Blood Pressure (JNC) classified patients according to blood pressure (**Table 6**).[3] Accordingly, when a patient's systolic blood pressure is greater than 140 or

Table 3
Clinical predictors of increased perioperative cardiovascular risk

Major	Unstable coronary syndromes
	Acute or recent MI
	Unstable or severe angina
	Decompensated heart failure
	Significant dysrhythmias
	High-grade atrioventricular block
	Symptomatic ventricular dysrhythmias
	Supraventricular dysrhythmias with uncontrolled ventricular rate
	Severe valvular disease
Intermediate	Mild angina pectoris
	Previous MI based on history or Q waves on ECG
	Compensated or previous heart failure
	Diabetes mellitus
	Renal insufficiency
Minor	Advanced age (>70 y)
	Abnormal result of ECG
	Rhythm other than sinus
	Low functional capacity
	History of stroke
	Uncontrolled systemic hypertension

Abbreviations: ECG, electrocardiogram; MI, myocardial infarction.

Data from Fleischer LA, Beckman JA, Brown LA, et al. American College of Cardiology/American Heart Association (ACC/AHA) 2007 Guidelines on perioperative cardiovascular evaluation and care for noncardiac surgery: a report of the American College of Cardiology/American Heart Association Task Force on Practice Guidelines. Circulation 2007;116:418–99.

diastolic blood pressure is greater than 90, pharmacologic treatment should be initiated.[4] Recently, the JNC released updates that described no change in classification, but rather stated specific targeted systolic and diastolic blood pressures and drugs based on gender, race, cardiac history, and other ongoing medical comorbidities.[4] Perioperatively, patients who have severe hypertension (>210/110 mm Hg) have an exaggerated hypotensive response to anesthesia and labile responses. Therefore, elective office surgery should be deferred if systolic blood pressure is greater than 180 and diastolic blood pressure is greater than 110 when other systemic comorbidities are present and if systolic blood pressure is greater than 210 and diastolic blood pressure is greater than 120 if no other comorbidities are present.[3]

Pacemaker/Defibrillator

Symptomatic bradycardia is treated with an implantable pacemaker.[5] A demand pacemaker discharges with missed beat or when heart rate is below a predetermined bradycardia threshold. A pacemaker can be single or dual chamber or biventricular where each ventricle is wired separately.[6] Recurrent ventricular tachycardia or ventricular fibrillation is treated with an implantable cardioverter-defibrillator (ICD). ICD is programmed to treat different dysrhythmias by defibrillating, cardioverting, or pacing. ICD provides a shock within 15 seconds of sensing a dysrhythmia.[7] When a patient has ICD and electrocautery will be used during an operation, the surgeon must communicate preoperatively with cardiology so that it is suspended intraoperatively and reprogrammed postoperatively. Alternatively, a magnet can be placed externally over the pacemaker to convert it to asynchronous mode.[8]

Coronary Artery Disease

Coronary artery disease (CAD) or atherosclerotic disease is defined as chronic inflammation of arterial endothelium by low-density lipoprotein, and lipid macrophage accumulation causes

Table 4
METs based on activities of daily living

Excellent (>7 METs)	Moderate (4–7 METs)	Poor (<4 METs)
Recreational sports (swimming, tennis, etc)	Cycling	Vacuuming
Jogging (10-min mile)	Walking 4 mph	Walking 2 mph
Household work (lifting furniture)	Light household work (dusting, dishes)	Personal care (dressing, eating, bathing)

Data from Fleischer LA, Beckman JA, Brown LA, et al. American College of Cardiology/American Heart Association (ACC/AHA) 2007 Guidelines on perioperative cardiovascular evaluation and care for noncardiac surgery: a report of the American College of Cardiology/American Heart Association Task Force on Practice Guidelines. Circulation 2007;116:418–99.

Table 5
Goldman criteria for cardiac index

Criteria	Points
History	
Age>70 y	5
Myocardial infarction<6 mo	10
Physical examination	
S3 gallop	11
Jugular venous distention	11
Aortic valve stenosis	3
Electrocardiogram	
Rhythm other than sinus or premature atrial contraction	7
>5 premature ventricular contractions per minute	7
General status	
Po_2<60 or Pco_2>50	3
K levels<3 mEq/L or HCO_3 levels<20 mEq/L	3
SUN>50 or creatinine>3 mg/dL	3
Abnormal AST or chronic liver disease	3
Bedridden	3
Operation	
Intraperitoneal, intrathoracic, aortic	3
Emergency	4

Abbreviations: AST, aspartate aminotransferase; SUN, serum urea nitrogen.
From Goldman L, Caldera DL, Nussbaum SR, et al. Multifactorial index of cardiac risk in noncardiac surgical procedures. N Engl J Med 1977;297:26.

atheromas and calcification of tunica medica, which leads to a narrowed artery with acute to chronic endothelial inflammation with an atheroma rupture or vasospasm. Risk factors for

Table 6
JNC classification

Category	SBP	DBP
Normal	<120	>80
Prehypertension	120–139	80–89
Stage I	140–159	90–99
Stage II	160–180	100–110
Urgent/ emergent	>180 With signs/ symptoms of end- organ damage	>110 Examples: rales, papilledema, headache, chest pain

Abbreviations: DBP, diastolic blood pressure; SBP, systolic blood pressure.
Adapted from James PA, Oparil S, Carter BL, et al. 2014 Evidence-based guideline for the management of high blood pressure in adults: report from the panel members appointed to the Eighth Joint National Committee (JNC 8). JAMA 2013;311(5):507–20.

CAD are male gender, increasing age, dyslipidemia, hypertension, diabetes, obesity, sedentary lifestyle, and family history.[9] Treatment consists of lifestyle modifications, pharmacologic therapy, and coronary revascularization.

Atrial fibrillation occurs when there is no coordinated electrical atrial conduction. The atrioventricular node sporadically reacts with no cardiac contraction, which reduces ventricular filling and cardiac output and places the patient at an increased risk for thromboembolic events. New atrial fibrillation is treated by electrical or pharmacologic cardioversion to obtain rate control. Patients are often placed on long-term anticoagulants such as Coumadin. The goal of Coumadin therapy is to maintain a balance between preventing clots and causing excessive bleeding. However, Coumadin has many drug interactions and a narrow therapeutic window and requires frequent monitoring. International normalized ratio (INR) provides information to prescribing physicians to ensure that Coumadin is producing the desired effect; it helps to ensure that the person's clotting time is at a therapeutic level without causing excessive bleeding or bruising.

ANTICOAGULATION

Newer oral anticoagulants were developed as alternatives to warfarin in the treatment of arterial and venous thromboembolism and in stroke prevention in patients with nonvalvular atrial fibrillation. These anticoagulants include dabigatran (Pradaxa), a direct thrombin inhibitor, as well as rivaroxaban (Xarelto) and apixaban (Eliquis), factor Xa inhibitors. These drugs do not require monitoring, and therefore patient compliance is essential. However, in emergency situations such as life-threatening bleeding or nonelective major surgery, they cannot be reversed because there are no antidotes currently available. Phase 1 and 2 research studies are ongoing.[10] For dabigatran, a specific antidote has been tested in a rat model of anticoagulation and a study in healthy male volunteers has been recently reported. For rivaroxaban, prothrombin complex concentrates (PCCs) have been found to completely reverse the prolongation of the prothrombin time induced by this new oral anticoagulant. For apixaban, recombinant factor VII was found in an experimental study using human blood to be superior to activated PCC and PCC.

The decision to discontinue anticoagulants should be based on the risk of surgical bleeding and discussion with the treating physician. For a simple procedure such as a single tooth extraction, there is typically no need to change these medications.[11] Local hemostatic measures suffice to control possible bleeding problems resulting from minor dental treatment. If multiple extractions are scheduled, after consultation with the prescribing physician, ideally, a patient should stop taking this medication 5 to 7 days before the scheduled procedure. If use of anticoagulants cannot be stopped because of the risk of thromboembolism, the patient's INR should be carefully monitored during the week before operation and obtained on the morning of the procedure. The desired range is 2 to 3, which often corresponds with the therapeutic range. There is no need to discontinue aspirin.[12] During surgical procedures involving high bleeding risk (multiple extractions, operations lasting>45 minutes, head and neck cancer surgery), the recommendation is to suspend the medication 2 to 3 days before the operation and consider bridging or switching to subcutaneous heparin or Lovenox.[13] Medication should be reintroduced after 24 hours, provided good hemostasis has been achieved.[14] The current idea for patients taking rivaroxaban (Xarelto), and apixaban (Eliquis) is to discontinue these medications, in the case of high surgical bleeding risk, 2 to 3 days before the procedure. Patients taking dabigatran (Pradaxa), with renal insufficiency and creatinine clearance between 30 and 50 mL/min, should discontinue the medication 2 to 4 days before the procedure.[15] Because of the rapid onset of action of these newer anticoagulant medications, bridging is reserved for patients with a high risk for thromboembolism and the inability to take oral medications for 2 or 3 days postprocedure.

ENDOCARDITIS PROPHYLAXIS

Valvular heart disease is a significant risk factor for perioperative complications. Valves can have stenosis or regurgitation. Mitral and aortic valve disorders are more common.[16] Conditions which require prophylaxis for endocarditis to include prosthetic heart valves, history of infective endocarditis, unrepaired cyanotic congenital heart disease, and repaired congenital heart defect with prosthetic material or device during the first 6 months following the procedure.[17] The antibiotic regimen remains the same and is given in **Table 7**.

MEDICATION-RELATED OSTEONECROSIS OF THE JAW

Management of patients with or at risk for MRONJ was discussed in the American Association of Oral and Maxillofacial Surgeons (AAOMS) position papers in 2007[18] and 2009.[19] Since then, the knowledge base and experience in addressing MRONJ has expanded, necessitating modifications and refinements to the previous guidelines.[20] A patient is considered to have MRONJ if all of the following criteria are met: current or previous treatment with antiresorptive or antiangiogenic agents, exposed bone or bone that can be probed through an intraoral or extraoral fistula in the maxillofacial region that has persisted for longer than 8 weeks, and no history of radiation therapy to the jaws or obvious metastatic disease to the jaws.[20] This new term was adopted to accommodate the growing number of osteonecrosis cases involving the maxilla and mandible associated with antiresorptive and antiangiogenic therapies. There are multiple hypotheses concerning the potential mechanisms leading to MRONJ, including altered bone remodeling, oversuppression of bone resorption, angiogenesis inhibition, constant microtrauma, suppression of innate or acquired immunity, vitamin D deficiency, soft tissue toxicity, inflammation, and/or infection.[20] Intravenous administration of medication increases the risk for MRONJ. The prevalence of osteonecrosis of the jaw increases over time. The risk of MRONJ

Table 7
Antibiotic prophylaxis for prevention of endocarditis

	Medication	Adults	Children
Oral	Amoxicillin	2 g	50 mg/kg
Allergic to penicillin	Clindamycin	600 mg	20 mg/kg
	Azithromycin	500 mg	15 mg/kg
Unable to take oral medicines	Ampicillin	2 g IM or IV	50 mg/kg IM or IV
Allergic to penicillin	Ceftriaxone	1 g IM or IV	50 mg/kg IM or IV
	Clindamycin	600 mg IM or IV	20 mg/kg IM or IV

Abbreviations: IM, intramuscularly; IV, intravenously.
Adapted from Wilson W, Taubert KA, Gewtiz M, et al. Prevention of infective endocarditis: guidelines from the American Heart Association: a guideline from the American Heart Association Rheumatic Fever, Endocarditis, and Kawasaki Disease Committee, Council on Cardiovascular Disease in the Young, and the Council on Clinical Cardiology, Council on Cardiovascular Surgery and Anesthesia, and the Quality of Care and Outcomes Research Interdisciplinary Working Group. Circulation 2007;116:1736–54.

in patients exposed to oral bisphosphonates (BPs) after tooth extraction is 0.5%.[21] The risk of MRONJ in patients exposed to intravenous BPs ranges from 1.6% to 14.8%.[20] The risk of developing MRONJ in patients who have been exposed to antiresorptive medications for dentoalveolar operations such as dental implant placement or endodontic or periodontal procedures is unknown.[20] Therefore, according to the special committee appointed by AAOMS, the risk of MRONJ after the above-mentioned procedures is comparable to the risk associated with tooth extraction.[20] Staging and treatment strategies are given in **Table 8**.

Table 8
Staging and treatment strategies for patients with MRONJ

Stage	Description	Treatment Strategies
At risk	No apparent necrotic bone in a patient who was treated with oral or intravenous BP	No treatment Patient education
Stage 0	No clinical evidence of necrotic bone but nonspecific clinical findings, radiographic changes, and/or symptoms	Systemic management (pain medication, antibiotics)
Stage 1	Exposed and necrotic bone or fistulas that probe to bone in patients who are asymptomatic and have no evidence of infection	Antibacterial mouth rinse, clinical follow-up on quarterly basis, patient education, review of indications for continued BP therapy
Stage 2	Exposed and necrotic bone or fistulas that probe to bone associated with infection as evidenced by pain and erythema in the region of exposed bone with or without purulent drainage	Symptomatic treatment with oral antibiotics, antibacterial mouth rinse, pain control, debridement to relieve soft tissue irritation, and infection control
Stage 3	Exposed and necrotic bone or a fistula that probe to bone in patients with pain, infection, and 1 or more of the following: • Exposed and necrotic bone extending beyond the region of alveolar bone resulting in pathologic fracture • Extraoral fistula • Oroantral or oronasal communication • Osteolysis extending to inferior border of mandible or sinus floor	Antibacterial mouth rinse, oral antibiotics, pain control, debridement or resection for longer-term palliation of infection and pain

Adapted from Ruggiero SL, Dodson TB, Fantasia J, et al. American Association of Oral and Maxillofacial Surgeons position paper on medication-related osteonecrosis of the jaw-2014 update. J Oral Maxillofac Surg 2014;72(10):1938–56; with permission.

SUMMARY

Patients who undergo oral and maxillofacial surgery are often relatively healthy, and complications related to medical conditions are not common. However, medical conditions may be present in any patient and may lead to increased morbidity and mortality unless these conditions are uncovered in those without such a history and recognized in those with a history of disease. A thorough medical and social history will elicit medical comorbidities when known. A thorough physical examination will often confirm the presence of systemic disease or identify it in those without a prior history.

Obtaining a thorough history and physical examination requires a systematic approach to a patient interview, consisting of: chief complaint, history of the chief complaint; a medical history with review of all systems, allergies, and medications, a social history, a family history, surgical history, and assessment of functional status. The sensitivity of a thorough history to identify a previously unrecognized medical condition should not be underestimated. The physical examination should also be standardized to include all relevant systems. The history and physical examination will then enable the surgeon to request additional investigations and medical referrals that allow risk stratification.

The risk assessment for each patient undergoing surgery requires an understanding of the surgical stress and the patient's medical condition. Major oral and maxillofacial surgery is considered to be intermediate in surgical operative risk. Oral and maxillofacial procedures performed in an ambulatory setting would be considered low risk.

Preoperative patient assessment is best completed by the surgeon who has a vested interest in the patient's well-being. When medical conditions and comorbidities are recognized preoperatively, appropriate workup or referral is easily organized. The involvement of other medical and surgical subspecialties should be readily sought when indicated. The ultimate goal of the preoperative evaluation is to identify medical concerns and provide the perioperative treatment algorithms that minimize patient morbidity.

REFERENCES

1. Fleischer LA, Beckman JA, Brown LA, et al. American College of Cardiology/American Heart Association (ACC/AHA) 2007 Guidelines on perioperative cardiovascular evaluation and care for noncardiac surgery: a report of the American College of Cardiology/American Heart Association Task Force on Practice Guidelines). Circulation 2007;116:418–99.
2. Goldman L, Caldera DL, Nussbaum SR, et al. Multifactorial index of cardiac risk in noncardiac surgical procedures. N Engl J Med 1977;297:26.
3. Matei V, Sami Haddadin A. Systemic and pulmonary arterial hypertension. In: Hines RL, Marschall KE, editors. Stoelting's anesthesia and co-existing disease. 6th edition. Philadelphia: Elsevier Saunders; 2012. p. 104–19.
4. James PA, Oparil S, Carter BL, et al. 2014 Evidence-based guideline for the management of high blood pressure in adults: report from the panel members appointed to the Eighth Joint National Committee (JNC 8). JAMA 2013;311(5):507–20.
5. Yew KL. Electrocution induced symptomatic bradycardia necessitating pacemaker implantation. Heart Views 2014;15:49–50.
6. Barol SS, Delnoy PP, Kucher A. Interventricular pacemaker-mediated tachycardia during biventricular pacing. Pacing Clin Electrophysiol 2014. [Epub ahead of print].
7. Joshi GP. Perioperative management of outpatients with implantable cardioverter defibrillators. Curr Opin Anaesthesiol 2009;22:701–4.
8. American society of anesthesiologist task force on perioperative management of patients with cardiac rhythm management devices. Practice advisory for the perioperative management of patients with cardiac implantable electronic devices: pacemakers and implantable cardioverter-defibrillators. An updated report by the American Society of Anesthesiologists Task Force on Perioperative Management of Patients with Cardiac Implantable Electronic Devices. Anesthesiology 2005;103:186–98.
9. Akshar S. Ischemic heart disease. In: Hines RL, Marschall KE, editors. Stoelting's anesthesia and co-existing disease. 6th edition. Philadelphia: Elsevier Saunders; 2012. p. 1–30.
10. Lévy S. Newer clinically available antithrombotics and their antidotes. J Interv Card Electrophysiol 2014;40:269–75.
11. van Diermen DE, Aartman IH, Baart JA, et al. Dental management of patients using antithrombotic drugs: critical appraisal of existing guidelines. Oral Surg Oral Med Oral Pathol Oral Radiol Endod 2009;107:616–24.
12. Servin FS. Is it time to re-evaluate the routines about stopping/keeping platelet inhibitors in conjunction to ambulatory surgery? Curr Opin Anaesthesiol 2010;23:691–6.
13. Mingarro-de-Leon A, Chaveli-Lopez B, Gavalda-Esteve C. Dental management of patients receiving anticoagulant and/or antiplatelet treatment. J Clin Exp Dent 2014;6:e155–61.
14. Spyropoulos AC, Douketis JD. How I treat anticoagulated patients undergoing an elective procedure or surgery. Blood 2012;120:2954–62.

15. Hankey GJ, Eikelboon JW. Dabigatran etexilate: a new oral thrombin inhibiter. Circulation 2011; 123:1436.

16. Herrera A. Valvular hear disease. In: Hines RL, Marschall KE, editors. Stoelting's anesthesia and co-existing diseases. 6th edition. Philadelphia: Elsevier Saunders; 2012. p. 31–47.

17. Nishimura RA, Carabello BA, Faxon DP, et al. ACC/AHA 2008 Guideline Update on Valvular Heart Disease: focused Update on Infective Endocardltis: a Report of the American College of Cardiology/American Heart Association Task Force on Practice Guidelines Endorsed by the Society of Cardiovascular Anesthesiologists, Society for Cardiovascular Angiography and Interventions, and Society of Thoracic Surgeons. J Am Coll Cardiol 2008;52: 676–85.

18. American Association of Oral and Maxillofacial Surgeons Position Paper on Bisphosphonate-Related Osteonecrosis of the Jaws. Advisory Task Force on Bisphosphonate-Related Osteonecrosis of the Jaws, American Association of Oral and Maxillofacial Surgeons. J Oral Maxillofac Surg 2007;65:369–76.

19. Ruggiero SL, Dodson TB, Assael LA, et al. American Association of Oral and Maxillofacial Surgeons position paper on bisphosphonate-related osteonecrosis of the jaws—2009 Update. J Oral Maxillofac Surg 2009;67(5 Suppl).2–12.

20. Ruggiero SL, Dodson TB, Fantasia J, et al. American Association of Oral and Maxillofacial Surgeons position paper on medication-related osteonecrosis of the jaw-2014 update. J Oral Maxillofac Surg 2014; 72:1938–56.

21. Kunchur R, Need A, Hughes T, et al. Clinical investigation of C-terminal cross-linking telopeptide test in prevention and management of bisphosphonate-associated osteonecrosis of the jaws. J Oral Maxillofac Surg 2009;67:1167–73.

Dental Extractions and Preservation of Space for Implant Placement in Molar Sites

Michael S. Block, DMD

KEYWORDS

- Dental implants • Extraction sites • Mandibular molars

KEY POINTS

- The algorithm for implant placement, either immediately after tooth removal or delayed, works well with excellent long-term crestal bone width maintenance.
- Clinicians can use tissue health as 1 factor to form their treatment strategy for the timing of implant placement into molar sites.
- Bone resorption is common after tooth extraction; the use of graft material may be necessary to provide ideal bone for implant placement and reconstruction of the patient with an esthetic and functional restoration.

INTRODUCTION

The clinician is often asked to remove a tooth and place an implant into the site. The implant must be placed with appropriate stability to allow for integration to occur, which requires bone presence. Bone is also necessary to allow for ideal implant positioning within the alveolus for functional and esthetic concerns. The purpose of this article is to discuss the changes in socket dimensions over time and how to promote space maintenance, with an algorithm for treatment based on evidence.

SOCKET HEALING

Socket healing approximates 40 days, beginning with clot formation and culminating in a bone-filled socket with a connective and epithelial tissue covering.[1,2] An extraction site may heal with bone formation to preserve the original dimensions of the bone. Unfortunately, bone resorption is common after tooth extraction. The use of graft material may be necessary to provide ideal bone for implant placement and reconstruction of the patient with an esthetic and functional restoration.

Bone resorption usually is greater in the horizontal plane than in the vertical plane.[3,4] Horizontal bone loss may be enhanced by thin facial cortical bone over the roots or bone loss from extension of local infection, such as caries or periodontal disease. Ideal placement of a dental implant centers the implant over the crest in a line connecting the fossae of the adjacent posterior teeth, or for anterior teeth, palatal to the emergence profile of the planned restoration. Unless the horizontal bone dimension is reconstructed or preserved after tooth extraction, implant placement is compromised, and in the esthetic zone, flattening of the ridge will occur, which results in a compromised restoration appearance. In the posterior mandible, these changes may be less dramatic, presumably because of the thickness of the buccal bone. The thin bundle bone, which was/is adjacent to the tooth roots, lies within the corpus of thick buccal cortical bone, and thus its remodeling may not result in rapid loss of ridge width.

Private Practice, 110 Veterans Memorial Boulevard, #112, Metairie, LA 70005, USA
E-mail address: DrBlock@cdrnola.com

Oral Maxillofacial Surg Clin N Am 27 (2015) 353–362
http://dx.doi.org/10.1016/j.coms.2015.04.001
1042-3699/15/$ – see front matter © 2015 Elsevier Inc. All rights reserved.

With regard to the esthetic zone of the maxilla, which includes the premolars, canines, and incisors, patients often present with teeth in need of extraction. Reasons for extraction of a single-rooted maxillary tooth in an adult include internal or external resorption after trauma, a breakdown of post and cores that were placed because of trauma, caries, root canal failure, and periodontal disease. Traditional protocols for restoring these sites rely on bone deposition to fill the extraction site before the implant is placed.[5,6] Hard and soft tissue grafting often is necessary to provide an ideal functional and esthetic restoration. Grafts compensate for the bone resorption that accompanies the natural healing process in an extraction socket.[7–10] When implants are placed 8–16 weeks after tooth extraction, the clinician must compensate for the loss of labial bone that occurs during the early phase of extraction site healing.[3,11,12] To prevent the need for hard or soft tissue grafting when implant placement is delayed, it is recommended to place an osteoconductive graft material within the extraction site to promote bone fill, to limit labial bone collapse, and to maintain bone for optimal implant placement.[13]

TREATMENT PLANNING

When a patient presents with a molar tooth in need of removal, 3 situations are common:

1. The tooth is nonrestorable but has intact surrounding bone and relatively healthy gingiva, with minimal pain (**Fig. 1**).
2. The tooth is nonrestorable and has intact surrounding bone. However, the tooth is acutely painful and may have purulent exudate and nonhealthy gingiva.
3. The tooth is nonrestorable but has lost a portion of the buccal bone (**Fig. 2**).

Preoperative imaging can determine the presence of the surrounding bone, the presence of interceptal bone, and the location of the inferior alveolar nerve canal in relation to the tooth. Sufficient space is necessary for placement of an implant of sufficient length to maintain a single molar implant tooth.

The molar tooth has roots that diverge and are separated by an isthmus of bone. The thickness of the bone between the roots may not be sufficient by itself for immediate implant placement. The labial and lingual cortical bone plates narrow in the apical regions and can be engaged to stabilize an implant in the molar site. The bone surrounding the molar tooth may be completely intact, or chronic infection may have caused large areas of bone loss, which if not grafted, result in inadequate bone available for implant placement. If the treatment plan includes placement of an implant into a posterior tooth site, cone-beam cross-sections

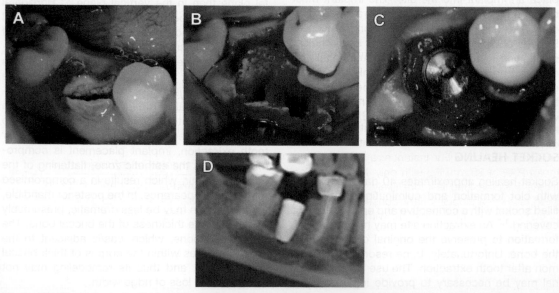

Fig. 1. (*A*) This patient required removal of a lower right first molar. The tooth was in cross bite. (*B*) A sulcular incision was made with vertical release sparing the papilla and a flap developed. The tooth was removed. (*C*) The implant was placed on the lingual aspect of the extraction site to correct the cross bite. The initial drill was placed without regard to interceptal bone, since the implant position needed to be different than the tooth's position due to the cross bite tendency. Allograft was placed into the defects from the root sockets. (*D*) A postoperative radiograph shows good implant positioning.

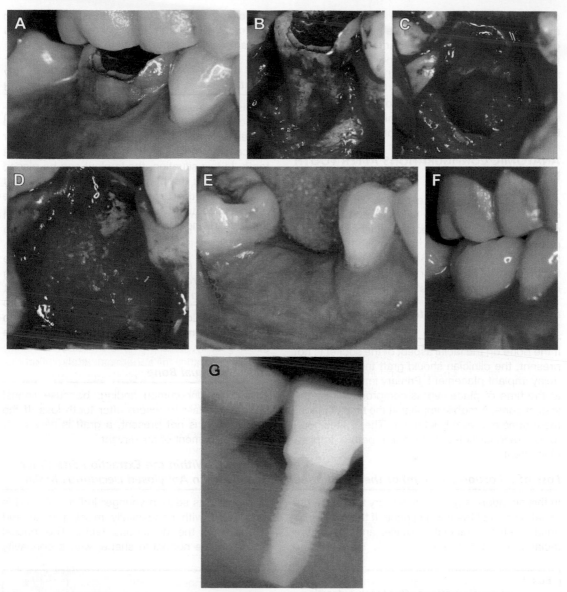

Fig. 2. (*A*) This patient's mandibular first molar requires extraction. The patient had been using antibiotics and chlorhexidine rinses preoperatively to reduce the bacterial flora around this tooth as much as possible. (*B*) An incision is made around the labial surface of the tooth and linked with 2 vertical extensions. The vertical releasing incisions are made within the site of the first molar, with care taken to avoid raising the attached tissues on the adjacent teeth. A full-thickness exposure is performed, exposing the lateral aspect of the tooth and the extensive bone loss. (*C*) The tooth is removed along with a small amount of granulation tissue. The area is irrigated thoroughly. Note the intact lingual plate of bone and the loss of the labial plate to the root apices. This defect has intact mesial and distal walls, as well as the lingual plate; therefore, this can be characterized as a 3-wall defect. (*D*) A graft of human mineralized bone is placed into the defect to reconstruct both the height and the width of the socket. After compaction of the graft material, the area is closed primarily. Primary closure was achieved with advancement of the keratinized gingiva, previously on the labial aspect of the tooth, and was sutured to the lingual aspect of the ridge. Chromic sutures are used in the vertical releasing incisions. To advance the flap, the periosteum was scored to provide mobilization of the flap, allowing tension-free closure. (*E*) 4 months later, the ridge has healed and is ready for implant placement. (*F*) This is the final crown 2 years after implant placement showing an excellent tissue response. (*G*) The 2 year radiograph showing excellent bone healing around the implant.

can be used to determine the amount of bone available or determine that there has been significant bone loss that prevents primary stability of the implant at time of tooth removal.[14] The technique described next has proved useful for grafting of the posterior molar site.

After reviewing the image from a cone beam scanner, and the physical examination of the patient, a decision can be made for treatment.

ANATOMIC CONFIGURATIONS AFTER TOOTH EXTRACTION

After a tooth has been extracted, the resultant defect in the bone may have several anatomic configurations that directly influence implant placement. This section discusses 10 findings that may be seen after tooth extraction. Each finding may be isolated or may be among several morphologic observations (**Box 1**).

Loss of All Facial Bone to the Apex of the Tooth

If the bone on the facial aspect of the socket is not present, the clinician should graft the socket and delay implant placement. Primary implant stability at the time of placement is compromised by the loss of bone. A mobile implant at the time of placement does not reliably integrate. These sites need to be reconstructed with bone before implant placement.

Loss of a Portion (3–6 mm) of the Facial Bone

In this situation, a graft is necessary to restore the facial portion of the missing bone. If the surgeon is unsure of the result in these cases and 50% of the facial bone has been lost as a result of the

pathology associated with the tooth, the preferred treatment is to graft the socket and place the implant 4 months after grafting.

Loss of Less Than 3 mm of Facial Bone at the Crest

This is a common situation when a tooth has extensive caries or a fracture. Crestal resorption may be limited to 3 mm from the planned gingival margin or the cemento-enamel junction (cej) of the adjacent tooth. In this situation, the implant can be placed at the level of the bone. This places the implant 3 mm from the gingival margin, which is the preferred location. There is usually no need to graft the buccal bone in this situation unless it is very thin.

Lack of Bone Inferior to the Apex of the Socket, with Extreme Proximity of Adjacent Vital Structures, Such as the Inferior Alveolar Canal or Mental Foramen

These extraction sites may need grafting prior to implant placement to ensure implant stability is achieved only.

Lack of Lingual Bone

This is an uncommon finding, because lingual bone is the last to resorb after tooth loss. If the lingual bone is not present, a graft is necessary before placement of an implant.

Concavity Within the Extraction Site When Removing an Ankylosed Deciduous Molar

This finding is seen in younger individuals and is associated with congenitally missing teeth and retention of the deciduous teeth. The buccal bone may be normal in shape, with a concavity

---

Box 1
Anatomic configurations after tooth extraction

1. Loss of all labial bone to the apex of the tooth
2. Loss of a portion (3–6 mm) of the labial bone
3. Loss of <3 mm of labial bone at the crest
4. Lack of bone superior to the apex of the socket, with extreme proximity of adjacent vital structures (eg, inferior alveolar canal, mental foramen, floor of the nose, floor of the sinus)
5. Lack of palatal or lingual bone
6. Concavity along the palatal or labial contours of the extraction site
7. Socket that is larger than the proposed diameter of the implant in all dimensions
8. Socket that is oval in shape, with the long dimension palatal to facial and the short dimension mesial to distal
9. Very thin surrounding bone
10. Bone adjacent to the neighboring tooth (or teeth) absent and root surface of adjacent tooth exposed

within the confines of the buccal and lingual cortical bone. These patients may have vertical deficiency and may need shorter implants with attention to avoid the inferior alveolar nerve.

A Socket That is Larger Than the Proposed Diameter of the Implant in all Dimensions

When an implant is placed into an extraction site, the normal drill sequence is used to prepare the implant site. Bone is removed until the implant can be placed and stabilized. When the diameter of the root of the tooth is larger than the implant in all dimensions, stabilizing the implant is most difficult unless bone is present beyond the apex of the socket or the cortical walls converge in the apical regions. In these cases, grafting of the large extraction socket provides the surgeon with an ideal site for placement of an implant after the graft has healed with bone formation in the socket.

Socket That is Oval in Shape, With the Long Dimension Palatal to Facial and the Short Dimension Mesial to Distal

The oval, or figure-eight–shaped, socket typically is found in canine or premolar sites, or within molar root sockets. The implant site is prepared in the ideal location to place the axis of emergence in the fossa or under the working cusp. After the implant has been placed, the gap between the implant and labial cortex can be grafted to prevent epithelial migration. The choice to graft or not to graft depends on the clinician; this author grafts the spaces in an attempt to promote bone formation and avoid epithelia migration.

Very Thin Surrounding Bone

After extraction of the tooth, the remaining facial bone may be exceptionally thin even when careful methods were used to preserve bone. In this situation, as long as the implant can be placed and secured in the surrounding bone, the implant can be placed, and the space between the implant and thin facial bone is grafted. If insufficient bone is present to stabilize the implants, a graft is indicated, and a delayed placement is planned. The thicker the labial plate, the greater the chance to maintain labial thickness.

Bone Adjacent to the Neighboring Tooth (or Teeth) Absent, and Root Surface of Adjacent Tooth Exposed

In this situation, the socket can be grafted, with the understanding that the final crestal bone level in the interdental area will be apical to the ideal position.

TREATMENT INDICATIONS IN 3 COMMON SITUATIONS

The Tooth is Nonrestorable but has Intact Surrounding Bone and Relatively Healthy Gingiva, with Minimal Pain

The tooth can be removed and an implant immediately placed. The indications for placement of an implant into a tooth site at the time of extraction include the following

1. Absence of purulent drainage
2. Healthy gingiva without gingival hyperplasia or erythema
3. Lack of active apical infection
4. Adequate bone present to allow ideal implant placement and stability

Reports indicate a high incidence of success in integration and function with implants placed immediately into extraction sites as long as the site has no purulent exudate, a healthy collar of gingival tissue is present around the tooth, and minimal lucency is seen at the apex of the tooth to be extracted.[15] The placement of implants into the extraction site immediately after tooth removal has been anecdotally recommended to eliminate an additional surgical procedure, prevent labial bone loss, and preserve the labial root form of the esthetic site.[16–23] Exposure of the implant into the oral cavity does not seem to result in a decrease in crestal bone levels.

Surgical procedure

After a conservative elevation of the gingiva to visualize the junction of bone to the tooth, the tooth is elevated gently and removed with minimal lateral subluxation. Every effort should be made to preserve the lateral cortical bone. As necessary, the tooth can be sectioned to facilitate bone preservation. Another option is to create a trough around the roots using the periotome insert for the Piezosurgery unit. The roots are easily removed after the Piezosurgery unit has been used. If present, granulation tissue is curetted. The site is irrigated gently with sterile saline, and the flap is tested to ensure passive rotation to the lingual tissues only to cover the root sockets on the mesial and distal aspect of the implant after implant placement.

A small round bur or bur of choice is used to locate a definitive hole in the bone exactly in the middle of the extraction site. This results in ideal restorative management. Placement of the implant asymmetrically in the extraction site leads to restorative problems. The sequencing drills are used to prepare the implant site as recommended for the specific implant used. This author finds that implants 5.0 mm or less in diameter may be difficult to achieve primary stability. Implants 5.4 to 6 mm in diameter are found to engage the cortical bone approximately 5 mm subcrestal and allow for excellent primary stability. Larger diameter implants may result in buccal bone thinning.

The implant is placed taking into consideration the level of the buccal and lingual bone and to avoid excessive countersinking. A healing abutment is placed. Allograft is usually used to graft the defects where the tooth roots had been. The gingiva is closed mesially and distally, leaving the healing abutment exposed. A large diameter healing abutment is recommended to allow for ease of abutment placement during the restorative phase after 4 months is allowed for integration.

The Tooth is Nonrestorable and has Intact Surrounding Bone; however, the Tooth is Acutely Painful and May Have Purulent Exudate and Non-healthy Gingiva

At the time of tooth extraction, the clinician may find purulent discharge, active periapical pathology, unhealthy gingiva with gingivitis and active periodontal disease in the mouth, a patient history of poor wound healing (eg, uncontrolled diabetes, chronic steroid use, immune compromise, alcoholism, drug dependence), or a lack of bone to stabilize an implant. In these cases, the tooth should be extracted and the implant placed after the infection and other local problems have resolved. In these situations, the implant can be easily placed 4 to 8 weeks after tooth removal into a noninfected and nonpainful site.

The surgical procedure is identical to the procedure described for immediate implant placement.

The Tooth is Nonrestorable but has Lost a Portion of the Buccal Bone

If there is loss of buccal bone, it is recommended to graft the site and proceed with implant placement after the bone has consolidated, typically 4 to 6 months after grafting. When the defect and socket are grafted with particulate material, the bone volume created and preserved depends on the density and retention of the graft within the socket. In contrast to single-rooted or premolar sites, which can be treated with a collagen plug over the socket, leaving the molar site open may result in loss of a portion of the graft. Therefore, primary closure is performed to retain the graft in molar sites. The incision design is critical for achieving primary closure of the site after placement of the graft.

The incision design allows advancement of the labial keratinized gingiva (KG) without advancement of the papilla and fixed gingiva on the adjacent teeth. The incision is made in the sulcus to within 2 mm of the interdental papilla. Vertical release incisions are made for full-thickness flap elevation to expose the lateral aspect of the alveolus and advance the flap to cover the site after graft material has been placed. When resorption of the labial or facial cortical bone has been extensive, elevation of the flap is performed with sharp dissection, with care taken to prevent perforation of the labial gingiva. After the flap has been raised, the periosteum is scored and relieved to allow passive advancement of the flap for primary closure.

Particulate graft material is placed into a small dish and dampened with sterile saline. A 1 mL plastic syringe can be used to deliver the graft. The tip of the syringe is removed with a scalpel and Rongeur forceps. The particulate graft is packed into the syringe and then placed into the extraction site. The graft material is compacted with a blunt instrument, and gauze is used to remove excess fluids. After the socket and bone defects have been restored to original form by the graft, the flap is advanced over the site.

A 4-0 chromic resorbable suture is used by the author to approximate the edge of the labial KG across the socket to the lingual gingiva. After the sutures have been placed, the vertical incisions are closed. Using this design, the labial KG is banked toward the lingual aspect of the ridge. It will be transposed to the labial surface of the abutment when the implant is placed. Occasionally, advancing the gingiva across the broad base of a maxillary molar is difficult. In this situation, a collagen material is placed over the palatal root site, and the buccal sockets are primarily closed with the KG, with sutures holding the collagen material in position similar to anterior sites (**Box 2**).

GRAFTING MATERIAL

The clinician should consider several points when choosing materials to graft the extraction socket:

1. Space should be maintained with a material that promotes bone incorporation and does not inhibit or adversely alter the normal sequence of extraction site healing.
2. The bone formed should be dense enough to allow stable placement of the implant. The material placed should have osteoconductive features to enhance bone formation.
3. The material should resorb within a selected period of time with replacement by bone that is normal to the site.
4. The resorption rate of the material over time should be taken into consideration to plan the

Box 2
Algorithm for implant placement after tooth removal

1. Buccal and lingual bone is intact. No purulent exudate; gingiva is healthy—remove tooth and immediately place implant if sufficient bone is available to stabilize the implant.

2. Buccal and lingual bone is intact. There is purulent exudate or the gingiva is not healthy—remove tooth and wait 4–6 weeks for resolution of the infection and then place the implant.

3. Buccal bone or intramedullary bone is not intact—remove tooth and place a graft. Close primarily. After 4 months place an implant.

sequencing of therapies such as implant placement, additional contour grafting, and pontic and site development.

5. The material should be relatively inexpensive, readily available, and should not transfer pathologic conditions.

BOVINE OR EQUINE SINTERED XENOGRAFT

Bovine or equine derived bone is a xenograft. It is a carbonate-containing apatite with crystalline architecture and a calcium/phosphate ratio similar to that of natural human bone.[24] With time, the sintered xenograft becomes integrated with bone. It may be slowly replaced by newly formed bone, but because the sintering process increases the crystallinity of the bone particles, it may not clinically appear to significantly resorb and will often be present years after placement.[24–27] When sintered xenograft material is used to graft an extraction site, 6 to –9 months may need to be allowed before placement of the implant. The relatively inert nature of this material delays revascularization and subsequent bone formation compared with more natural materials such as autogenous bone.[28,29]

MINERALIZED BONE ALLOGRAFT

Human mineralized bone in particulate form can result in short-term preservation of an extraction site's bone bulk and volume in preparation for the placement of implants. The advantages of an allograft are (1) the graft material is readily available without the need for a second surgical harvest site, and (2) the material is osteoconductive. Over time, the allograft resorbs, and, it is hoped, replaced with bone.

Human mineralized bone is available as particulate cortical or cancellous bone. The recommended particle size ranges from is 250 μm to 1.0 mm. Allografts are prepared by bone banks. Sterile procedures are used to harvest the bone, which is washed with a series of delipidizing agents such as ethers and alcohol, lyophilized, and then sieved to the particle size necessary for

a specific indication. The freeze-dried mineralized bone allograft usually is irradiated to sterilize it even though the entire process for harvesting to packaging is performed under strict sterile conditions. Comparative reports and clinical results involving different methods of processing mineralized bone are limited. The choice of allograft should be based on the ease of delivery, cost, consistency in the appearance of the graft material, and quality of the bone bank.

When placed in an extraction site, mineralized bone graft material is still present at 4 months.[30] However, the bone forming around the mineralized bone particles usually is sufficiently mineralized to allow immediate provisionalization, with adequate primary stability after placement of the implant in the extraction site grafted with a mineralized allograft.

One goal of grafting of the extraction site is retention and preservation of the original ridge form and maintenance of the crestal bone after the implants have been restored. In 1 study in which no membrane was used at the time of extraction site grafting, the grafted sites felt bone hard at 4 months and appeared to be filled with bone.[10] The average mesial crestal bone level was −0.66 plus or minus 0.67 mm (range, 0 to −1.27 mm) at implant placement and 0.51 plus or minus 0.41 mm (range, 0−−1.91 mm) at final restoration. The average distal crestal bone level was −0.48 plus or minus 0.68 mm (range, 0.64−−1.91 mm) at implant placement and 0.48 plus or minus 0.53 mm (range, 0–1.27 mm) at final restoration. A measurement of 1.27 mm from the top of the shoulder of the implants correlated to the level of the first thread of the implant.[30] Bone heights were maintained with mineralized bone graft material.

AUTOGENOUS BONE

Clinicians believe that the ideal bone replacement graft material has always been autogenous bone.[31–34] Few clinicians use a separate harvest site to obtain autogenous bone to graft extraction sites. The past use of bone harvested from the symphysis, ramus, or maxillary tuberosity is not a common, current procedure. Bone removed during alveoloplasty can be used as a graft. Bone can be scraped from adjacent sites, collected in a sieve after the bone has been shaved with a bur and collected with Rongeur forceps from adjacent sites or the alveolar ridge.[35]

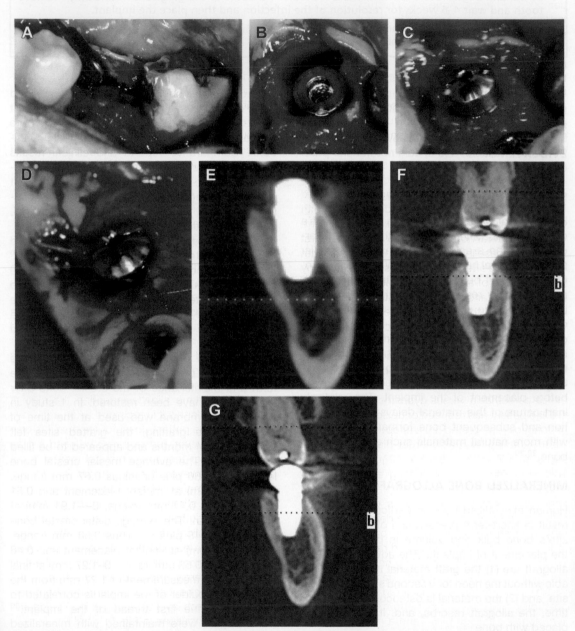

Fig. 3. (*A*) This patient had the first molar removed and the site grafted secondary to a large abscess form a fractured tooth. He recently fractured the lingual cusp to the level of the alveolar bone and is planned for tooth removal and immediate implant placement. (*B*) The tooth was removed and the implant placed in the middle of the socket, through the interceptal bone. The radiofrequency index was 82, indicating excellent primary stability. (*C*) Allograft was placed into the sockets. (*D*) The healing abutment was placed, and the mesial and distal gingiva were gently approximated to the lingual. (*E*) This is the immediate postplacement cross section radiograph. (*F*) 5-year follow-up cross section of the grafted first molar site, showing excellent maintenance of the crestal width. (*G*) 5-year follow-up cross section of the immediate placement second M site, showing excellent maintenance of the crestal width, compared with **Fig. 3**E.

POSTOPERATIVE CARE

The patient is given antibiotics and pain medication. Antibacterial rinses are not used after graft placement because of toxicity to fibroblasts and other cells involved with epithelialization. The patient is given instructions for a soft diet to avoid trauma from chewing textured food on the surgical site.

The sutures are removed 7 to 10 days after graft placement. A cone beam collimated 6 cm scan is taken 3 months after graft placement for evaluation of the bone height for implant placement. Implants are usually placed 4 months after graft placement.

EVIDENCE FOR LONG-TERM PRESERVATION OF BONE

The following are preliminary data form an Institutional Review Board (IRB)-approved retrospective evaluation with 4- to 5-year follow-up on crestal width changes after tooth removal and implant placement (Block and Scogin, unpublished data, 2014). Three groups were evaluated with 4- to 5-year follow-up cone beam scans after implant placement and restoration. Patients with mandibular molars to be removed with implant placement were included. Three groups were measured. One group had the tooth removed and an implant immediately placed. A second group had the molar tooth removed and the implant placement 4 to 10 weeks after tooth removal. The third group had buccal bone loss that required grafting with implant placement 4 to 6 months after tooth removal.

The width of the crestal bone from facial to lingual was measured. Intraexaminer error on multiple measures was determined to be 0.3 mm. The width of the ridge at the crest, 5 mm, and 10 mm inferior to the crest was measured prior to tooth removal, at the time of implant placement, and at long-term follow-up (**Fig. 3**).

The results showed

1. No changes in width measurements 5 and 10 mm inferior to the crest for any time period for any group.
2. The width of the ridge at the crest decreased from 1 to 1.5 mm over the 4- to 5-year period of time.
3. These changed were statistically significant compared with pre-extraction and implant placement time periods.
4. There were not significant width changes in the early time periods from extraction to the implant placement time period, only the long-term time period.

From this preliminary set of data, there appears to be excellent maintenance of crestal width at the implant shoulder region, regardless of the timing of implant placement.

SUMMARY

The algorithm for implant placement, immediately after tooth removal or delayed, works well, with excellent long-term crestal bone width maintenance. Clinicians can use tissue health as 1 factor to form their treatment strategy for the timing of implant placement into molar sites.

REFERENCES

1. Amler MH, Johnson PL, Salman I. Histological and histochemical investigation of human alveolar socket healing in undisturbed extraction wounds. J Am Dent Assoc 1960;61:32–44.
2. Amler MH. The time sequence of tissue regeneration in human extraction wounds. Oral Surg Oral Med Oral Pathol 1969;27:309–18.
3. Lekovic V, Kenney EB, Weinlaender M, et al. A bone regenerative approach to alveolar ridge maintenance following tooth extraction: report of 10 cases. J Periodontol 1997;68:563–70.
4. Lekovic V, Camargo PM, Klokkevold PR, et al. Preservation of alveolar bone in extraction sockets using bioabsorbable membranes. J Periodontol 1998;69:1044–9.
5. Nir-Hadar O, Palmer M, Soskolne WA. Delayed immediate implants: alveolar bone changes during the healing period. Clin Oral Implants Res 1998;9:26–33.
6. Palmer RM, Smith BJ, Palmer PJ, et al. A prospective study of astra single tooth implants. Clin Oral Implants Res 1997;8:173–9.
7. Block MS. Hard and soft tissue grafting for esthetic implant restorations. In: Babbush C, editor. Dental implants: the art and science. Philadelphia: Saunders; 2000. p. 217–28.
8. Block MS, Salinas TS, Finger IM, et al. Incidence of hard and soft tissue grafts in esthetic maxillary implant restorations. J Oral Maxillofac Surg 2000; 58(8 suppl 1):77.
9. Gher ME, Quintero G, Assad D, et al. Bone grafting and guided bone regeneration for immediate dental implants in humans. J Periodontol 1994;65:881–91.
10. Tritten CB, Bragger U, Fourmousis I, et al. Guided bone regeneration around an immediate transmucosal implant for single tooth replacement: a case report. Pract Periodontics Aesthet Dent 1995;7:29–38.
11. Gruber H, Solar P, Ulm C. Maxillomandibular anatomy and patterns of resorption during atrophy. In: Watzek G, editor. Endosseous implants: scientific and clinical aspects. Chicago: Quintessence; 1996. p. 29–60.

12. Lang N, Becker W, Karring T. Alveolar bone formation. In: Lindhe J, editor. Textbook of clinical periodontology and implant dentistry. 3rd edition. Copenhagen (Denmark): Munksgard; 1998.

13. Block MS. Soft tissue esthetic procedures for teeth and implants. In: Block MS, Sclar T, editors. Atlas of the oral and maxillofacial surgery clinics. Philadelphia: Saunders; 1999. p. 61–78.

14. Nedir R, Bischof M, Szmukler-Moncler S, et al. Predicting osseointegration by means of implant primary stability. Clin Oral Implants Res 2004;15: 520–8.

15. Arlin ML. Immediate placement of osseointegrated dental implants into extraction sockets: advantages and case reports. Oral Health 1992;82(19–20):23–4, 26.

16. Mazor Z, Peleg M, Redlich M. Immediate placement of implants in extraction sites of maxillary impacted canines. J Am Dent Assoc 1999;130:1767–70.

17. Rosenquist B, Grenthe B. Immediate placement of implants into extraction sockets: implant survival. Int J Oral Maxillofac Implants 1996;11:205–9.

18. Schwartz-Arad D, Chaushu G. Placement of implants into fresh extraction sites: 4 to 7 years retrospective evaluation of 95 immediate implants. J Periodontol 1997;68:1110–6.

19. Werbitt MJ, Goldberg PV. The immediate implant: bone reservation and bone regeneration. Int J Periodontics Restorative Dent 1992;12:206–17.

20. Grunder U, Polizzi G, Goené R, et al. A 3-year prospective multicenter follow-up report on the immediate and delayed immediate placement of implants. Int J Oral Maxillofac Implants 1999;14:210–6.

21. Schwartz-Arad D, Grossman Y, Chaushu G. The clinical effectiveness of implants placed immediately into fresh extraction sites of molar teeth. J Periodontol 2000;71:839–44.

22. Wohrle PS. Single-tooth replacement in the aesthetic zone with immediate provisionalization: fourteen consecutive case reports. Pract Periodontics Aesthet Dent 1998;10:1107–14.

23. Gomes A, Lozada JL, Caplanis N, et al. Immediate loading of a single hydroxyapatite-coated threaded root form implant: a clinical report. J Oral Implantol 1998;24:159–66.

24. Berglundh T, Lindhe J. Healing around implants placed in bone defects treated with Bio-Oss: an experimental study in the dog. Clin Oral Implants Res 1997;8:117–24.

25. Artzi Z, Tal H, Dayan D. Porous bovine bone mineral in healing of human extraction sockets. Part 1. Histomorphometric evaluations at 9 months. J Periodontol 2000;71:1015–23.

26. Wetzel AC, Stich H, Caffesse RG. Bone apposition onto oral implants in the sinus area filled with different grafting materials: a histologic study in beagle dogs. Clin Oral Implants Res 1995;6:155–63.

27. van Steenberghe D, Callens A, Geers L, et al. The clinical use of deproteinized bovine bone mineral on bone regeneration in conjunction with immediate implant installation. Clin Oral Implants Res 2000;11: 210–6.

28. Block MS, Kent JN. A comparison of particulate and solid root forms of hydroxylapatite in dog extraction sites. J Oral Maxillofac Surg 1986;44:89–93.

29. Block MS, Kent JN. Healing of mandibular ridge augmentations using hydroxylapatite with and without autogenous bone in dogs. J Oral Maxillofac Surg 1985;43(1):3–7.

30. Block MS, Finger I, Lytle R. Human mineralized bone in extraction sites before implant placement: preliminary results. J Am Dent Assoc 2002;133:1631–8.

31. Becker W, Urist M, Becker BE, et al. Clinical and histologic observations of sites implanted with intraoral autologous bone grafts or allografts: 15 human case reports. J Periodontol 1996;67:1025–33.

32. Robinson E. Osseous coagulum for bone induction. J Periodontol 1969;40:503–10.

33. Schallhorn RG, Hiatt WH, Boyce W. Iliac transplants in periodontal therapy. J Periodontol 1970; 41:566–80.

34. Froum SJ, Thaler R, Scopp IW, et al. Osseous autografts: I. Clinical responses to bone blend or hip marrow grafts. J Periodontol 1975;46:515–21.

35. Gunther KP, Scharf H-P, Pesch H-J, et al. Osseointegration of solvent preserved bone transplants in an animal model. Osteologie 1996;5:4–12.

Managing Impacted Third Molars

Louis K. Rafetto, DMD

KEYWORDS

• Third molars • Asymptomatic • Disease free • Retention • Management strategies

KEY POINTS

- Clinicians can be reasonably certain about some, but not all, things related to the behavior of third molars.
- There is a tangible, measurable, but not totally predictable risk for future extraction among patients with retained third molars that were asymptomatic and disease free at the time of baseline examination.
- Based on an analysis of relevant historical, clinical, and imaging information, findings can be organized based on the presence or absence of symptoms and disease, which helps simplify decision making.
- Oral and maxillofacial surgeons should educate their patients and the community about the benefits and consequences (short and long term) of different third molar management strategies, including active surveillance.

One of the most common decisions made by oral and maxillofacial surgeons is how best to manage third molars. Most of these decisions are straightforward owing to the presence of symptoms and/or disease. Recently these decisions have come under increased scrutiny. Commonly cited areas of concern include when surgical management is indicated (particularly in the case of asymptomatic teeth), the optimal timing for treatment, the cost of treatment, and what should be done when a decision is made to retain a third molar.

There are differences of opinion when it comes to what constitutes best practice in the area of third molar management. In an effort to develop consensus on best-practice approaches to any clinical dilemma, attention should be given to evidence-based clinical practice and its role in the decision-making process. This process is characterized by merging the best available evidence (ideally from practice-based research) with the results of a comprehensive and focused clinical

and imaging examination. As a result, recommendations can be made to the patient.

This article reviews what is known about third molar behavior and advocates an organized approach to the clinical problem. Such an approach begins with the collection of relevant clinically generated data followed by review of this information in light of what is known about the behavior of third molars. The last part of the process is formulation of a management strategy with implementation after an informed discussion.

OBSTACLES TO CONSENSUS

As is the case in many areas of clinical practice, some clinicians may disagree with any proposed management strategy.

DESIRES AND PERSPECTIVES OF PARTIES OF INTEREST

Patients and families focus their attention on risks, convenience, and limiting out-of-pocket

Department of Oral & Maxillofacial Surgery & Hospital Dentistry, Christiana Care Health System, 3512 Silverside Road, Suite 12, Wilmington, DE 19810, USA
E-mail address: lkrafetto@gmail.com

Oral Maxillofacial Surg Clin N Am 27 (2015) 363–371
http://dx.doi.org/10.1016/j.coms.2015.04.004
1042-3699/15/$ – see front matter © 2015 Elsevier Inc. All rights reserved.

expenses and red tape. Clinicians value the freedom to provide what they think is the best treatment and to be fairly compensated. Third parties and government agencies focus on cost management and quality measures. Consumer groups and media outlets focus on risks of operative treatment and the potential for overtreatment. This lack of unanimity in part represents honest disagreement but also reflects the bias of self-interest (**Fig. 1**).

Uncertain Terminology

"Asymptomatic" does not indicate the absence of disease, but merely the absence of symptoms. It is well understood that disease precedes symptoms and that disease often progresses in the absence of symptoms. Effective management strategies should take into account the likelihood of the development of disease.

Misconceptions

In the eyes of many clinicians, third molar decision making consists of either tooth removal or retention. Management may also include partial removal (coronectomy), retention with active clinical and radiographic surveillance, surgical exposure, tooth repositioning, transplantation, surgical periodontics, and marsupialization of associated soft tissue disorder with observation and possible secondary treatment.

Unlike medicine, the dental profession in the United States is made up of about 80% general practitioners, with most of the remaining 20% practicing in disciplines other than surgery. Most patients seeking consultation have been referred from other different dental professionals who have nothing at stake other than the well-being of the patient.

RELATED ORGANIZATIONAL POLICY STATEMENTS

Several professional organizations have developed policy statements on third molar management.

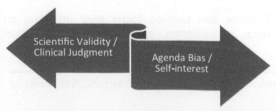

Fig. 1. Agenda bias and self-interest are obstacles to arriving at the best care.

American Association of Oral and Maxillofacial Surgeons

The American Association of Oral and Maxillofacial Surgeons[1] (AAOMS) "Parameters of Care 2012: Clinical Practice Guidelines for Oral and Maxillofacial Surgery (ParCare 2012)" lists more than 20 specific indications for removal of categories of third molars along with goals for therapy. It recognizes the benefit of removal to prevent disease and the role of the treating surgeon as the person best qualified to determine care for an individual patient. Therapeutic goals listed include "prevention of pathology," "preservation of periodontal health of adjacent teeth," and "optimization of prosthetic rehabilitation." Along with specific indications are the following statements: "Given the following and the desire to achieve therapeutic goals, obtain positive outcomes, and avoid known risks and complications, a decision should be made before the middle of the third decade to remove or continue to observe third molars knowing that future treatment may be necessary based on the clinical situation. There is a growing body of knowledge suggesting that retention of third molars that are erupted or partially erupted contribute to a higher incidence of periodontal disease. This persistent periodontal disease has both dental and medical consequences for the host and therefore, may be an indication for prophylactic removal."[1]

The AAOMS also offers so-called anchor statements, best represented by the following: "Predicated on the best evidence-based data, impacted teeth that demonstrate pathology, or are at high risk of developing pathology, should be surgically managed. In the absence of pathology or significant risk of pathology, active clinical and radiographic surveillance is indicated."

The American Dental Association

The American Dental Association offers statements that are less detailed but support in principle the guidelines contained in the AAOMS ParCare document. Comments include that, "Your dentist or specialist may also recommend removal of teeth to prevent problems or for others reasons, such as…" "In addition, the condition of your mouth changes over time. Wisdom teeth that are not removed should continue to be monitored, because the potential for developing problems later on still exists. As with many other health conditions, as people age, they are at greater risk for health problems and that includes potential problems with their wisdom teeth."

Academy of Pediatric Dentistry

The Academy of Pediatric Dentistry advocates for the removal of asymptomatic third molars if there is a likelihood of future disease. In addition, "When a decision is made to retain impacted third molars, they should be monitored for change in position and/or development of pathology, which may necessitate later removal."[2]

Cochrane Systematic Review

"General agreement exists that removal is appropriate in case of symptoms of pain or pathological conditions. Controversial statements exist with regard to the prophylactic removal of asymptomatic or disease-free impacted third molars. This review found no evidence to support or refute routine prophylactic removal of asymptomatic impacted wisdom teeth in adults; no studies of adults met the criteria for inclusion."[3]

United Kingdom's National Health Service

The UK National Health Service (NHS) restricts the removal of third molars based on recommendations issued by the National Institute of Clinical Evidence (NICE) in an effort to restrain short-term costs. "The routine practice of prophylactic removal of pathology-free impacted third molars should be discontinued in the NHS" and "Surgical removal of impacted third molars should be limited to patients with evidence of pathology. Such pathology includes unrestorable caries, nontreatable pulpal and/or periapical pathology, cellulitis, abscess and osteomyelitis, internal/external resorption of the tooth or adjacent teeth, fracture of tooth, disease of follicle including cyst/tumour, tooth/teeth impeding surgery or reconstructive jaw surgery, and when a tooth is involved in or within the field of tumour resection."[4]

In a recent article, McArdle and Renton[5] reviewed the effects of the NICE guidelines and concluded that third molar removal is now as common as it was before their institution. The investigators state that the dynamics of removal have altered with the changing mean age of patients, and that the reason for extraction is now predominantly caries, periodontal disease, and pericoronitis rather than impaction.[5]

National Health Service of Finland

The National Health Service of Finland has a policy similar to the NICE guidelines, despite a highly regarded Finnish researcher having published data from a long-term retention study documenting that most patients who retain their third molars eventually have 1 or more removed based on the development of disease. Further, their methodology allows many patients with retained third molars to have associated disease even if overtly asymptomatic.[6]

United States Military

The US Military supports removal of third molars based on the findings/recommendation of the treating surgeon. Appointees to the military academies are required to have their third molars removed before entrance in recognition of the benefits of prophylactic treatment.

American Public Health Association

In 2008, the American Public Health Association (APHA) issued a policy statement opposing the prophylactic removal of wisdom teeth.[7] This policy was not based on an evidence-based analysis or formulated with the benefit of input from experts in wisdom tooth management. It was formulated by a long-time critic well known for his bias against removal of third molars. This policy treats all third molar extractions as unnecessary and extrapolates isolated cost and complication data to imply great financial impact. It lacks consideration of active surveillance as well as the costs associated with ignoring the long-term effects on local (and possibly systemic) health and quality of life.

Approaches like those of the APHA and NICE emphasize the outcomes of third molar removal but overlook the costs and outcomes associated with retention, because that is where most of the available data are.

THIRD MOLARS ARE DIFFERENT

Third molars are different from other teeth in important ways, highlighted by their greater frequency and severity of disease and because they are typically nonfunctional. Important differences are, to a large degree, secondary to their location as the most distal teeth in the dental arch, and they are the last to erupt into the oral cavity, leaving less physiologic space for eruption and maintenance. The resulting poor-quality soft tissue support often leads to percolation of bacteria beneath the gingival tissues surrounding the third molar, contributing to subclinical inflammation that often progresses to pericoronitis and infection (**Fig. 2**). Periodontal pocketing is frequently found around third molars, as well as dental caries, which are difficult to restore. In addition, the roots of these teeth, particularly with increasing age, are more likely to approximate important anatomic structures such as the maxillary sinus, adjacent teeth, and the neurovascular canal, as well as

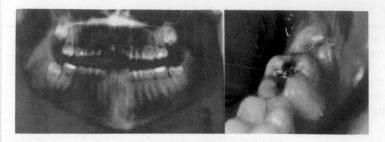

Fig. 2. Despite #17 near occlusal plane, it lacks physiologic space for eruption and maintenance.

being positioned in places where associated infections may become more of an issue because of the position of the mylohyoid muscle and thin area of the lingual cortical plate, which can predispose to bacterial migration to adjacent facial spaces, leading to deep facial space infections. Removal may therefore be the most cost-effective path and allow a healthier oral environment.

CLINICALLY RELEVANT SCIENCE

Considerable evidence published over the last decade has moved clinicians closer to answering important questions about third molars. As in all matters of decision making, relevant evidence should be fairly interpreted by those who are expert, experienced, and active in the management of patients with third molars, using an organized approach to evaluate the validity and clinical relevance of evidence (**Fig. 3**).

Highlights include a series of prospective, longitudinal studies conducted by investigators from a variety of disciplines at multiple sites known as the Third Molar Clinical Trials. This effort resulted in more than 125 articles and abstracts published in peer-reviewed journals. Also important was the 2010 AAOMS Multidisciplinary Conference on Third Molar Science.[8] Experts from the United States, Canada, Finland, and the United Kingdom presented and reviewed the latest research findings on third molar extraction, retention, patient surveillance, potential risks, and attendant costs. Many other articles have been published since these efforts and have helped to give better clarity to what is known and what needs further study.

As a result, there is general agreement on important aspects of third molars and their behavior.

KNOWN ASSOCIATED DISEASE

There are well documented disorders associated with retained third molars. These include but are not limited to:

1. Caries
2. Pericoronitis
3. Root resorption
4. Periodontitis
5. Infections (local and fascial space)
6. Cysts (**Fig. 4**)
7. Tumors
8. Mandible fractures

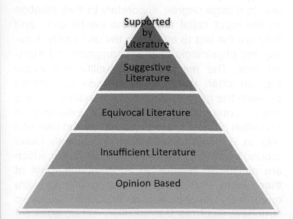

Fig. 3. Hierarchy of clinically relevant evidence.

Supported by Literature

Suggestive Literature

Equivocal Literature

Insufficient Literature

Opinion Based

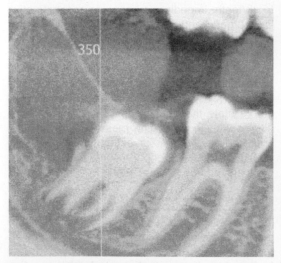

Fig. 4. Second molar unable to erupt (contralateral molar erupted) because of odontogenic cyst at unformed third molar site.

POTENTIAL ADVERSE OUTCOMES ASSOCIATED WITH THIRD MOLAR REMOVAL

As with any form of treatment, complications may occur secondary to any management approach, including retention. Complications from third molar removal are generally minor and resolve within a few days. Problems that may be associated with the removal of third molars include inflammatory complications, such as infection or osteitis; hemorrhage; injury to adjacent anatomic structures, teeth, or nerves; periodontal defects; fractures of maxillary tuberosity or mandible; persistent oral-antral communication; retained roots; and the need for additional treatment to manage complications. The risks and implications of third molar retention are less well documented, but are equally important.

CONSEQUENCES OF THIRD MOLAR RETENTION

Recently the AAOMS established a committee of experts to address an important clinical question: among young adults who elect to retain their asymptomatic third molars, what is the risk of having 1 or more third molars extracted in the future?[0] They conducted a systematic review of the literature. During the initial search, 65 articles were identified that reported on patients who required extraction of previously asymptomatic third molars. Seven articles met inclusion criteria for the final analysis. Studies included were prospective, had sample sizes greater than or equal to 50 subjects with at least 1 asymptomatic third molar, and at least 12 months of follow-up. The annual and cumulative incidence rates of third removal were estimated.

The mean incidence rate for the extraction of previously asymptomatic third molars was 3.0% per year with the cumulative incidence rates for removal ranging from 5% at 1 year to 64% at 18 years. The reasons for extraction were predominantly caries, periodontal disease, and other inflammatory conditions. The group concluded that the cumulative risk of third molar extraction for young adults with asymptomatic third molars is sufficiently high to warrant discussion when reviewing the risks and benefits of third molar retention as a management strategy.

In light of the findings discussed earlier, and given that the absence of symptoms does not equal the absence of disease, it is clear that patients who elect to retain their third molars should be followed with active surveillance, including recommendations for the frequency of regular follow-up visits.

Note that clinicians who support retention as a lower cost option fail to consider these lifetime risks associated with third molar retention and should factor in the current and future costs of active surveillance and risks of incurring the costs of treatment, which can range from the full scope of restorative options to extraction on either a planned or unplanned basis.

It is clear that, despite most patients eventually requiring removal of their third molars, some are able to maintain them for a lifetime (although some are nonfunctional). However, at this time, it cannot be determined with confidence what the future will be for all patients with asymptomatic disease-free teeth. Accordingly, it comes down to the clinicians' ability to use experience and expertise to develop a sense of the likelihood of disease developing and to communicate that in realistic terms to the patient. In the case of a decision to retain, a reasonable interval between follow-up for patients is every 2 years, and sooner if symptoms or obvious signs become evident (**Fig. 5**).

THINGS CONSIDERED CERTAIN ABOUT THIRD MOLAR BEHAVIOR AND MANAGEMENT

1. Third molars are different from other teeth in significant ways.
2. An absence of symptoms associated with third molars does not equate to the absence of disease.
3. Retained wisdom teeth frequently and unpredictably change position, eruption, and periodontal status.
4. The microbial biofilm associated with partially erupted third molars and pericoronitis is conducive to the development of periodontal disease.
5. Periodontal disease in the third molar area begins with their eruption.
6. Pocketing around wisdom teeth is an important indicator of periodontal disease, especially when bleeding occurs on probing.

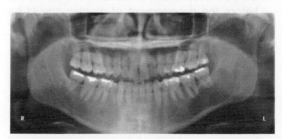

Fig. 5. Keratocyst identified on image of 34-year-old patient with unexplained tingling in his lower lip. He returned to his dentist as a part of active surveillance of his retained third molars.

7. Third molars with probing depths greater than 4 mm increase the risk for developing increased pocketing anteriorly.
8. Extraction of a third molar reduces the risk for periodontal disease in young adults.
9. There are identifiable risk factors for delayed healing and for surgical complications associated with third molar surgery.
10. There are identifiable ways to improve postoperative healing and recovery.
11. Most patients with retained, asymptomatic, disease-free wisdom teeth eventually require surgical management.
12. When patients elect to retain their third molars, the frequency of future disease is sufficiently high that active surveillance is a superior management strategy compared with symptomatic (as needed) follow-up.

STATEMENTS LIKELY TO BE VALID BUT REQUIRING MORE STUDY BEFORE BEING CONSIDERED CERTAIN

1. Although it is likely that most third molars will develop disease over time, clinicians are not certain how to identify those that can be maintained.
2. Active surveillance of retained wisdom teeth may be more expensive than extraction in the long term.
3. Some clinicians suggest that systemic diseases are linked to the oral inflammation associated with third molars. Although this may be true, and although it does make biological and clinical sense, current evidence for a cause-and-effect link is suggestive rather than definitive.

RECOMMENDATIONS SUPPORTED BY CLINICALLY RELEVANT EVIDENCE

1. Surgical management of third molars is appropriate when there is evidence of disease.
2. Surgical intervention or removal of third molars before the development of disease should be considered in patients who have insufficient physiologic space for eruption and maintenance at a time when the postsurgical healing is optimal and the risk of complications low (**Fig. 6**).
3. To limit the known risks and complications associated with surgery, it is medically appropriate and surgically prudent to remove third molars in patients with demonstrated disease before the middle of the third decade and before complete root development.
4. Given that third molars have been shown to be dynamic in their behavior and position, patients

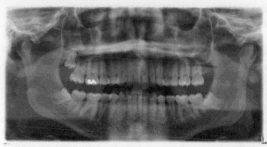

Fig. 6. A 28-year-old patient who previously elected retention of asymptomatic third molars. Roots approach inferior alveolar nerve and clinical findings include increased periodontal pockets at distal side of second molars. Removal is now more likely to be associated with prolonged recovery, possible complications, and increased cost associated with advanced imaging to assess position of root tips in relation to nerve.

choosing to monitor them are committed to a lifetime of follow-up. The known variables of active surveillance include the cost of regular imaging and follow-up visits, the uncertainty regarding the future behavior of the teeth, the risk for developing inflammatory dental disease, and a statistically significant increased risk with age for operative or postoperative complications if extraction or other treatment becomes unavoidable.
5. Third molars that are completely erupted and functional, symptom free, free of caries, in hygienic position with a healthy periodontium, and without other associated pathologic conditions do not require extraction, but do require routine maintenance and periodic clinical and radiographic surveillance.
6. An impacted tooth with completed root formation that is totally covered by bone in a patient beyond the third decade that is not associated with disease should be monitored for change in position and/or development of disease, which may then indicate its removal.

SIMPLIFIED APPROACH TO CLINICAL DECISION MAKING

Although the recommendations discussed earlier provide guidelines in the best management of patients with third molars, there is no formula that can be applied successfully to answer every clinical question about the best management of wisdom teeth.

Where there is evidence of disease, management is generally straightforward. When symptoms are present, it is important to identify the source with subsequent management focused on removal or control of the cause.

Uncertainty is more prominent in the case of patients who have asymptomatic disease-free third molars. Common sense dictates that the optimum strategy should be somewhere between removal of all versus retention of all. Given that clinicians cannot confidently predict what the future holds for all patients with asymptomatic disease-free teeth, they must rely on the clinician's ability to use experience and expertise in developing a sense of the likelihood that disease will develop and communicate this in realistic terms to the patient.

A helpful way to take what is known about third molar behavior and apply it to the clinical setting has been advocated by Dodson.[10] This strategy involves categorizing teeth based on the presence of symptoms (S+) or absence of symptoms (S−) as well as the presence of disease (D+) or absence of disease (D−).

This approach begins with a thorough medical and dental history with attention paid to any symptoms that may be associated with the wisdom teeth. Often patients do not report overt symptoms, whereas others may have vague complaints. The clinician should ascertain whether they are related to their third molars or whether they are from another source. In part, this is done through clinical and radiographic examinations.

Physical examination should include eruption status and position of the tooth in the jaws/oral cavity, functionality, and periodontal and caries status. Imaging allows determination of the presence or absence of the tooth, presence or absence of disease, anatomy of the tooth and its root system, as well as its relationship to important structures such as the inferior alveolar nerve, adjacent second molar, and maxillary sinus. In addition, imaging can detect significant associated (and nonassociated) disorders, such as cysts or tumors.

Teeth are then categorized into (1) symptomatic and disease present (S+/D+), (2) symptomatic and disease absent (S+/D−), (3) asymptomatic and disease present (S−/D+), and (4) asymptomatic and disease absent (S−/D−). In general, the largest category of patients presenting to oral and maxillofacial surgery offices is S−/D+ (about half), followed by S−/D− (about a third), with the smallest category being S+/D− (less than 1%).

SYMPTOMS AND DISEASE PRESENT

Patients in the first group (S+/D+) generally present with pain, swelling, and/or trismus. Common findings include acute pericoronitis, dental caries, bone loss, localized or fascial space infection, or a combination (**Fig. 7**). Treatment should focus on

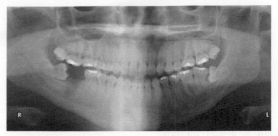

Fig. 7. Patient who is S+/D+.

addressing the presence of disease, with removal of the offending third molar as the preferred treatment strategy. In some cases, dental restoration, periodontal therapy, and/or enhanced hygiene may be considered based on the patient's ability to maintain adequate hygiene, the restorative status of the tooth, its functional usefulness, and the desires of the patient. If damage has occurred secondary to the disease process, attention should also be directed to repair any defect.

SYMPTOMS PRESENT/DISEASE FREE

Patients in the S+/D− group are seen less frequently than those in other groups. If symptoms are secondary to impending tooth eruption, the surgeon must decide whether it is likely to erupt into a useful position. Other times the symptoms are not related to the third molars and may represent myofascial disorders or odontogenic disease of nearby teeth (**Fig. 8**). Management is based on the likelihood of developing associated disease and the functionality of the third molars, particularly if the surgeon is unable to identify the source

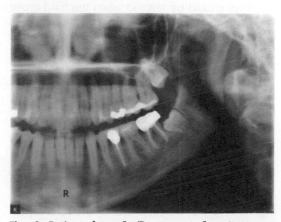

Fig. 8. Patient from S+/D− group. Symptoms are caused by an unresolved disorder from #18. Treatment options may include retreatment of #18 with removal of #17 (inadequate physiologic space/interference with restoration of #18), or removal of #18 to allow possible eruption and repositioning of #17.

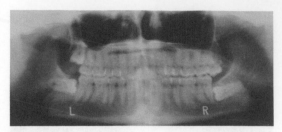

Fig. 9. S−/D+ patient.

of symptoms. The patient and family should be informed of the uncertainty of resolving symptoms if they cannot be directly linked to the third molars.

SYMPTOM FREE/DISEASE PRESENT

Patients in the this group, S−/D+, typically present with periodontitis, dental caries, or a cyst or tumor associated with the tooth. Treatment focuses on removal of disease and its cause, with options favoring removal. Other possible options include restoration, periodontal therapy, and enhanced hygiene (**Fig. 9**). Here again, if damage has occurred secondary to the disease process, attention should be directed to repair if possible.

SYMPTOM FREE/DISEASE FREE

This group, the least straightforward and most controversial, consists of patients with no current symptoms or disease (S−/D−) (**Fig. 10**). In the absence of evidence to support routinely retaining or removing third molars in this group, the surgeon should review the likelihood of disease developing in the future, functionality, risks of removal, risks of retention, and protocol for active surveillance. Removal should be favored when the third molar is or is likely to be nonfunctional, when there is an overlying removable prosthesis, when the

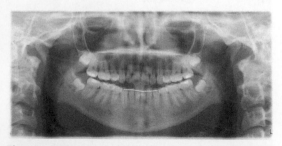

Fig. 10. A 16-year-old girl with unerupted and asymptomatic third molars. Clinical examination is necessary to help ascertain physiologic space for eruption and maintenance. Informed discussion should include potential consequences of surgical management as well as consequences of retention and the impact of age on risks.

removal for orthodontic removal is justified (such as when the tooth is preventing the eruption of the second molar), and in the case of planned orthognathic surgery. Patients should also be informed of the greater difficulty and increased rate of complications with removal of wisdom teeth as they age. When appropriate, patients should be told that, if they retain their disease-free wisdom teeth, it is possible that they will live their entire lives without problems.

SUMMARY

Based on extensive evidence, oral and maxillofacial surgeons can be certain, or reasonably certain, about important aspects of the behavior of wisdom teeth and the outcomes of different management strategies.

A recent article documents a tangible, measurable, but not totally predictable risk for future extraction among patients with retained third molars that were asymptomatic and disease free at the time of baseline examination. Although the annual risk is low, the cumulative lifetime risk is considerably higher, with most teeth requiring operative management over time. When patients elect to retain a third molar, they should be advised about this risk of removal over time. Given the increased complication rate when third molars are removed with increasing age, it may be more prudent to extract them by the middle of the third decade.

In the pursuit of a model for best practice, this knowledge should be applied to the clinical setting by surgeons who are expert, experienced, and active in providing care for patients with third molars. Where there is an absence of conclusive evidence, the available evidence should be interpreted in a manner that is most likely to benefit the patients, considering both short-term and long-term consequences of removal and retention strategies. An organized approach based on the patient's symptom and disease status is useful in simplifying management recommendations.

ACKNOWLEDGMENTS

The author acknowledges Alexandra C. Rafetto for her contributions to this article.

REFERENCES

1. American Association of Oral and Maxillofacial Surgeons. Parameters of care: clinical practice guidelines for oral and maxillofacial surgery (AAOMS ParCare 2012), dentoalveolar surgery version 5.0 DEN 1. J Oral Maxillofac Surg 2012.

2. American Academy on Pediatric Dentistry Council on Clinical Affairs. Guidelines on pediatric oral surgery. Pediatr Dent 2014;30(7 Suppl):205–11.

3. Mettes TG, Nienhuijs ME, van der Sanden WJ, et al. Interventions for treating asymptomatic impacted wisdom teeth in adolescents and adults. Cochrane Database Syst Rev 2005;(2):CD003879.

4. National Institute of Clinical Excellence (N.I.C.E.) on the indications for the removal of third molars. 2000. Available at: nice.org.uk.

5. McArdle L, Renton T. The effects of NICE guidelines on the management of third molar teeth. Br Dent J 2012;213:E8.

6. Ventä I, Ylipaavalniemi P, Turtola L. Long-term evaluation of estimates of need for third molar removal. J Oral Maxillofac Surg 2000;58:288.

7. Opposition to prophylactic removal of third molars (wisdom teeth). Policy date: 10/28/2008, policy number: 20085. 2008. Available at: apha.org.

8. Dodson TB, Rafetto LK, Nelson WJ. Introduction. Proceedings of the Third Molar Multidisciplinary Conference. Washington, DC, October 19, 2010. J Oral Maxillofac Surg 2012;70(9):S2–3.

9. Bouloux GF, Busaidy KF, Beirne OR, et al. What is the risk of future extraction of asymptomatic third molars? A systematic review. J Oral Maxillofac Surg 2014. [Epub ahead of print].

10. Dodson TB. The management of the asymptomatic, disease-free wisdom tooth: removal versus retention. Atlas Oral Maxillofac Surg Clin North Am 2012;20:169–76.

Coronectomy
Partial Odontectomy or Intentional Root Retention

M. Anthony Pogrel, DDS, MD, FRCS

KEYWORDS

- Coronectomy • Intentional root retention • Partial odontectomy • Third molars • Wisdom teeth
- Inferior alveolar nerve

KEY POINTS

- Coronectomy protects the inferior alveolar nerve from damage when lower third molars need removing.
- Cone-beam computed tomography (CBCT) has become the standard of care in deciding whether to offer coronectomy to a patient where there is a close relationship between the tooth and the nerve.
- There are reported variations in technique, but they do not seem to affect the results.
- Root migration seems to be the most frequent complication.

My personal interest in coronectomy started when I heard Brian O'Riordan (a London-based oral and maxillofacial surgeon) give his retirement talk to the annual meeting of the British Association of Oral and Maxillofacial Surgeons in Buxton, England in 1997. The title of his talk was "Uneasy Lies the Head that Wears a Crown."[1] In this he presented a fascinating story of his 30-year love affair with coronectomies and showed much of the rationale and also his long-term results. I returned to California energized and determined to try this technique. At that time, it was not widely practiced in the United States and nobody was lecturing or publishing on the topic. As we began to develop the technique and look at our early results (our first publication was in 2004),[2] the technique began to gain some popularity locally and nationally, and although it still remains controversial in the United States, it did assume a degree of respectability when the American

Dental Association approved a procedure code (D7251) for coronectomy, effective January 2011. However, just because the American Dental Association recognized the technique and gave it a code number does not make it universally accepted and even more does not ensure that dental insurance companies will reimburse for the technique, and even now several of them do not reimburse for this technique. Nevertheless, the technique does seem to be gaining wider acceptance, although there are some differences in the indications and actual technique used within and between countries.

In this article I discuss these differences in the light of personal experience. The degree of acceptance of the technique in some ways can be judged on the number of articles in peer-reviewed journals on the topic. From 1965 to 2004, there were only seven articles on coronectomy in the English language literature over a 38-year period,[1,3–8] and all

Department of Oral and Maxillofacial Surgery, University of California San Francisco, Box 0440, Room C522, 521 Parnassus Avenue, San Francisco, CA 94143-0440, USA
E-mail address: tony.pogrel@ucsf.edu

Oral Maxillofacial Surg Clin N Am 27 (2015) 373–382
http://dx.doi.org/10.1016/j.coms.2015.04.003
1042-3699/15/$ – see front matter © 2015 Elsevier Inc. All rights reserved.

of these were after 1988. Since then, the numbers each year are as follows:

2004	3
2005	3
2006	2
2007	1
2008	1
2009	5
2010	5
2011	6
2012	8
2013	11
2014	6

CONTROVERSIAL ISSUES CONCERNING CORONECTOMY

Most authorities agree that the technique is indicated when there is high probability of damage to the inferior alveolar nerve if the whole tooth is removed. Previously evaluations were made on Panorex radiographs using several criteria including overlapping of the nerve shadow on the roots of the teeth, narrowing of the nerve shadow, or deviation of the nerve shadow.[9–12]

Although medical-grade (also called fan beam or multislice) computed tomography (CT) scanning has been available since the mid-1970s to determine the relationship in three dimensions, it was not widely used because it was relatively expensive, the radiation dosage was comparatively high, the availability was limited, insurance would not reimburse for it, and the software did not allow easy visualization of the relationship between the inferior alveolar nerve and the roots of the third molar. The increasing availability of cone-beam CT (CBCT) scanning from 2002 onward eased these problems in that the radiation dose is much lower than with fan-beam CT, the cost is much lower (around $300 in the United States), and the software makes easy visualization of the relationship between the inferior alveolar nerve and the tooth in three dimensions. CBCT scanning is now the preferred imaging technique to determine in three dimensions what appears to be a close relationship between the inferior alveolar nerve and the third molar roots.[13–19]

Classifications of the relationship of the nerve to the tooth vary on CBCT, but in general there are three groups, based on the risk of permanent inferior alveolar nerve damage following removal of the whole tooth.

1. Low risk: This occurs when the panoral radiographic appearance turns out on the CBCT scan to be superimposition only. There is separation of the nerve and the root with a covering of bone in between (**Fig. 1**).
2. Medium risk: This occurs when the nerve is directly adjacent to the roots of the tooth or is mildly grooving the root of the tooth (**Fig. 2**).
3. High risk: This occurs when there is deep grooving of the tooth by the nerve or even perforation of the tooth root by the nerve with the roots growing around the nerve (**Fig. 3**).

We prefer not to use numbers, or percentages, because patients often want to apply overall numbers to their own personal situation.

It is important to realize the differences in image acquisition with fan-beam (medical grade) CT and CBCT scanning. In principle, fan-beam or medical-grade CT uses slices that are now usually less than 1 mm apart, to build up a composite image. In contrast, CBCT scanning uses volumetric image acquisition and visualization. Because of this, the resolution of CBCT scanning cannot match that of fan-beam CT scanning and so it is not always possible to visualize the exact relationship at some

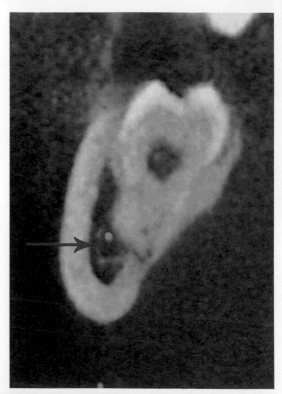

Fig. 1. A coronal slice from a cone-beam CT scan showing the inferior alveolar nerve (*arrow*) as separate from the root of the tooth. This represents a low risk of permanent nerve involvement following removal of the tooth.

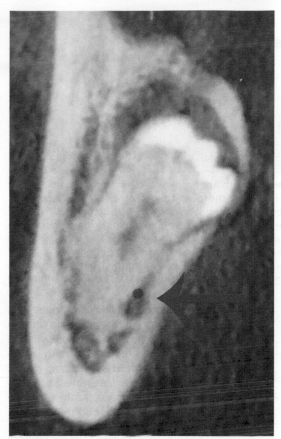

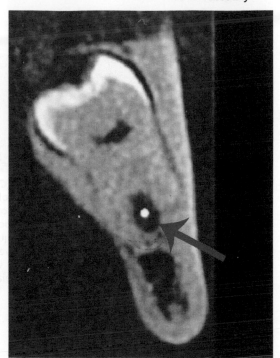

Fig. 3. A coronal slice of a cone-beam CT scan showing the inferior alveolar nerve (*arrow*) passing between the roots of the lower third molar. This represents a high risk of permanent nerve involvement should this tooth be removed in one piece.

Fig. 2. An axial slice of a cone-beam CT scan where the inferior alveolar nerve (*arrow*) is directly adjacent to the root of the tooth and is lightly grooving it. There is no indication of cortical bone separating the nerve from the tooth. This represents a medium risk of permanent nerve involvement following removal of the tooth.

precise points. The images shown in **Fig. 4** are of a case where the nerve actually passed through a hole in the roots, and although a CBCT scan was taken preoperatively, the resolution did not allow direct visualization of the root perforation. Therefore, this tooth was subsequently removed complete and the perforation was seen clinically. If this had been accurately visualized preoperatively, it is likely that a coronectomy would have been performed.

INDICATIONS FOR CORONECTOMY

The technique is generally performed on lower third molars but occasionally on deeply impacted second molars and even very occasionally first molars.[20] The technique is offered to any patient when there is a moderate or high risk of damage to the inferior alveolar nerve if the tooth is removed completely as assessed by Panorex-type radiograph supplemented by CBCT scanning. The technique may be offered in low-risk cases on patients older than 25 or where nerve involvement might present special problems (eg, wind

instrument players). The patient's age is important in treatment planning, in that conceptually coronectomy is believed to be more appropriate for older patients, who in general do not tolerate nerve damage as well as young patients. It was not initially designed for teenagers (the commonest group having third molars removed in the United States) for the following reasons:

1. It is often important to remove the tooth completely in teenagers in conjunction with orthodontic treatment.
2. Teenagers are less likely to get nerve involvement because the nerve is more resilient.
3. If they do get nerve involvement, it is more likely to recover and less likely to result in permanent dysesthesia.
4. Even if it does turn out to be permanent in a teenager, they often get used to it and are hardly aware of it, whereas older patients are much less adaptable and much more likely to be inconvenienced by the discomfort of permanent nerve involvement.

In our particular program, we do not routinely offer coronectomy to younger patients having third molars removed unless it is believed that they are at medium or high risk. For older patients, it is offered even when there is a low risk.

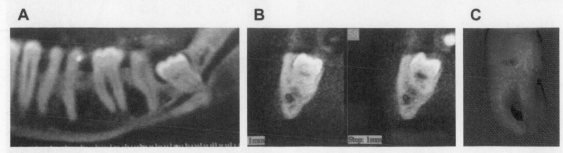

Fig. 4. (*A*) Panoramic reconstruction. (*B*) Axial slices. (*C*) Actual tooth after removal. These represent an attempt to visualize the relationship between the inferior alveolar nerve and the lower third molar before tooth removal. The cone-beam CT, because of its more limited power of resolution, cannot visualize objects in the detail that can be obtained with fan-beam CT. In this case, the cone-beam CT scan was unable to show that the nerve went right between the roots of the tooth. The tooth was consequently removed without coronectomy, but fortunately the mesial root fractured and so it was possible to remove the tooth without causing permanent nerve damage. If this had been visualized preoperatively, coronectomy would probably have been performed. (*From* Pogrel MA. Coronectomy to prevent damage to the inferior alveolar nerve. Alpha Omegan 2009;102:61–7; with permission.)

CONTRAINDICATIONS FOR CORONECTOMY

The following situations are contraindications for coronectomy:

- When the tooth is lying horizontally along the path of the inferior alveolar nerve. In these circumstances, sectioning of the crown could present as high (if not higher) risk of nerve involvement than just taking out the whole tooth (**Fig. 5**).
- Where it is not believed that all the enamel of the tooth can be removed. Retention of enamel seems to be associated with a much higher failure rate (**Fig. 6**).
- Infection involving the roots of the teeth.
- Caries involving the roots of the teeth.
- If the roots are mobilized during the procedure, they should be removed.
- When the second molars are to be distalized orthodontically.

SURGICAL TECHNIQUE

As the procedure has gained wider acceptance the numbers of variations on the basic surgical technique have increased. As originally conceived, the technique involved total sectioning of the crown of the tooth, removal of all enamel, and removal of enough of the coronal portion of the tooth such that the portion to be retained was at least 2 to 3 mm below the alveolar crest of bone. This was believed to be important for new bone to grow over the retained roots and for them not to become exposed. As described by our unit, the technique involves raising buccal and lingual flaps, the placement of a lingual retractor to protect the lingual nerve and lingual soft tissues so that the crown of the tooth could be sectioned with a 702-type fissure bur through the whole crown of the tooth.[2] This is the technique that is still used in our unit (**Fig. 7**). However, two other techniques have been described.

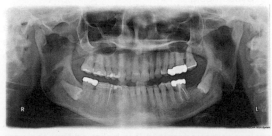

Fig. 5. Lower third molars lying horizontally along the inferior alveolar nerve making it impossible to carry out coronectomy.

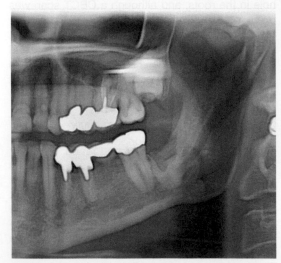

Fig. 6. A postcoronectomy radiograph showing retained enamel on the mesial aspect of the lower left third molar.

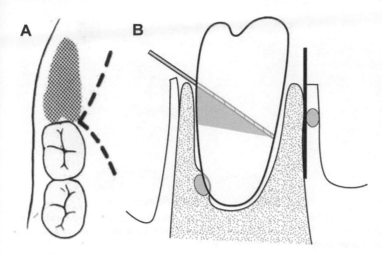

Fig. 7. (*A*) The conventional third molar incision extending down the external oblique ridge to the disto-buccal line angle of the lower second molar with a buccal releasing incision going no further forward than the midpoint of the first molar to avoid a frequent arteriole located in this area. (*B*) Diagramatic representation of coronectomy technique. A lingual retractor has been placed to protect the lingual soft tissues, including the lingual nerve, and a 702 fissure bur is used at approximately a 45-degree angle to section the crown completely before removal. The *gray area* represents the portion of the tooth root that is then removed to place them 3 to 4 mm below the alveolar crest. (*From* [A] Pogrel MA. Partial odontectomy. Oral Maxillofac Surg Clin North Am 2007;19:85–9, with permission; and [B] Pogrel MA, Lee JS, Muff DF, et al. Coronectomy: a technique to protect the inferior alveolar nerve. J Oral Maxillofac Surg 2004;62:1447–52, with permission.)

The first is a similar technique except that a lingual flap is not raised and a lingual retractor is not placed, but rather the crown of the tooth is removed from above with either a fissure bur or a high-speed round bur such that the crown is either split vertically from above into small sections or it is just ground away until one ends up 2 to 3 mm below the alveolar crest.

The second is a technique whereby no lingual flap is raised and no lingual retractor is used, but the crown is still sectioned horizontally in the same manner as one would use for routine third molar removal. In this, the fissure bur is taken approximately two-thirds of the way across the tooth and then the crown is fractured off in the normal way with a straight elevator. The crown is then removed and the roots smoothed if necessary to the correct level.[21] In this technique there is a reasonable possibility of mobilizing the retained roots, which must then be removed. However, the proponents of this particular technique state if the roots are mobilized or loosened, it normally means that the nerve could not be too intimately involved with the roots and therefore they can be removed without undue risk. If the roots are firm, they are retained in the usual way. Studies using this technique always show a higher incidence of failed coronectomies in that the roots are removed at the initial surgery. However, proponents of this technique do not report any higher incidence of inferior alveolar nerve involvement.

Coronectomy can also be used in conjunction with removal of pathology in the third molar region.

The most frequent instance of this is in the case of the dentigerous cyst (**Fig. 8**). Although a fairly large defect may be left, this does not seem to require any type of grafting in most cases.[22] No authors currently recommend any type of endodontic treatment of the retained roots,[23] and articles have shown that the retained roots do remain vital.[24]

Other areas showing differences in techniques are discussed next.

Antibiotics

Many authors have always believed that the use of antibiotics is important for the success of this technique. It is believed that antibiotics should be given prophylactically so that they are in the pulp chamber of the tooth to be sectioned at the time of removal. This means giving them perioperatively if given intravenously, or an hour preoperatively if given orally. However, several authors have published on carrying out the technique without using any antibiotics, and the success rates and infection rates seem similar.[21,25–27]

Suturing

In our technique we raise a buccal flap, and undermine and release the periosteum if necessary, to obtain a tension-free, water tight, primary closure of the socket.[28] This was believed to be important for primary healing and for new bone to grow over the socket. However, some authors suture without raising a buccal flap and without periosteal release, so that the socket is not completely closed.[21] Again, success rates seem to be similar.

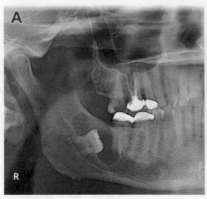
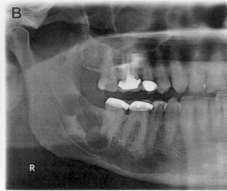

Fig. 8. Radiographs demonstrating the technique being used in the presence of pathology. (*A*) Preoperative image showing an impacted lower right third molar in a close relationship with the inferior alveolar nerve and associated with a dentigerous cyst. (*B*) Postcoronectomy.

The Distance Below the Alveolar Crest to Leave the Roots

As originally described, this technique recommended removal of the tooth until it was 2 to 3 mm below the alveolar crest of bone (**Fig. 9**). These numbers were derived from animal studies, primarily in dogs.[29–31] Now that there are adequate results obtained from clinical studies on patients, it does seem that the technique works best if the retained roots are left 3 to 4 mm below the alveolar crest of bone.[15,25,32] By leaving them a little lower down, the bone grows over the roots more consistently and they may move somewhat less.

RESULTS

Randomized controlled clinical trials are difficult to perform but have been attempted[33,34] as have case control studies.[15] Other studies are mainly case series[2,25,35–37] or review articles.[38,39] Most published papers describe successful results with a low complication rate.[32] Because the technique is designed to avoid permanent damage to the inferior alveolar nerve, most published papers do show that this aim is achieved.[28,35,40,41]

Typically the infection rate is noted to be no higher than with complete third molar removal, and by definition there can be no dry socket because there really is no socket. Most cases of infection seem to result from leaving some enamel behind, from the tooth being removed. There seems no doubt that retained enamel can harbor bacteria and that bone does not attach to enamel, leaving a potential problem area.

Excessive pocketing behind the second molar has not been reported, and on average, pocket depths measure 2 to 4 mm. If this is believed to be an issue grafting has been suggested.[42]

The major complication seems to be that many of these roots subsequently migrate. Migration occurs at different times but can be visible on radiographs 3 months after the extraction. It appears as a periapical radiolucency and comparison of serial Panorex radiographs makes the movement obvious (**Fig. 10**). Some practitioners have

Fig. 9. Clinical result postcoronectomy. Note the exposed pulp chamber and the retained root fragments below the rim of the alveolar crest. (*From* Pogrel MA, Lee JS, Muff DF, et al. Coronectomy: a technique to protect the inferior alveolar nerve. J Oral Maxillofac Surg 2004;62:1447–52; with permission.)

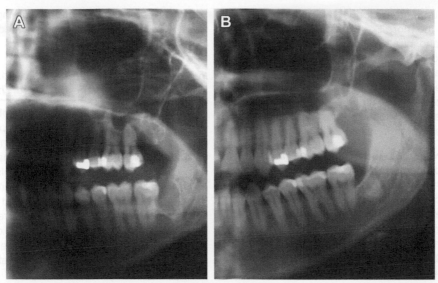

Fig. 10. Panorex radiographs showing early migration of retained roots of lower left third molar. (*A*) Immediately postcoronectomy. (*B*) Four months later. Note that beneath the apices of the roots there is a radiolucency that has been mistaken for periapical infection. Roots have moved despite the appearance of bone growing over the roots.

mistaken the periapical radiolucency for infection, but this is not the case. The radiolucency merely represents the space where the roots were but have now migrated. The roots always appear to migrate away from nerve, and although sometimes they do migrate all the way to the surface (**Fig. 11**), they seem to be easy to remove without complication and this may occur in 1% to 5% of cases.[21,43] It was believed that if the nerve truly perforated the roots, or the roots were deeply grooving them, they could not in fact migrate. However, cases have been described where the roots have migrated apically taking the inferior alveolar nerve up with them.[3] Obviously, if roots such as these had to be removed subsequently, considerable care would need to be taken.

In our own program, the results are as follows:

- Total number of cases carried out between 1997 and August 2014: 742.
- Infections: six (0.8%); two roots subsequently required removal.
- Number of teeth migrating following coronectomy: 230 (31%).
- Number of roots subsequently requiring removal: six or 0.8% (two for infection and four because of migration). One of these patients suffered an inferior alveolar nerve injury (see later).
- The number of teeth migrating and the number of retained roots that are subsequently removed is probably related to the time of

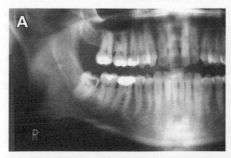
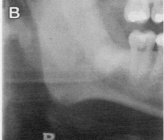
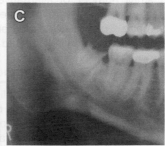

Fig. 11. Radiograph showing coronal migration of the retained roots of a lower third molar over a 2-year period. (*A*) Preoperative appearance showing gross decay of the tooth. (*B*) Six months postcoronectomy showing good healing with apparent bone over the retained roots. (*C*) Two years postcoronectomy showing occlusal migration of the retained root necessitating removal now without risk to the inferior alveolar nerve. (*From* Pogrel MA. Coronectomy to prevent damage to the inferior alveolar nerve. Alpha Omegan 2009;102:61–7; with permission.)

follow-up, and the longer the patients are followed, the more likely it is that retained roots move and need removal. We need to await 20- and 30-year follow-up studies to assess the final outcome.
- Number of failed coronectomies (roots were mobilized at the time of surgery and were removed): 12, none causing inferior alveolar nerve symptoms.

In our own series, the infection rate is actually lower for coronectomy than for routine third molar removal, and we have speculated on the reason for this. It could simply be that many of our third molars are removed by residents in training, whereas coronectomies are normally performed by attendings, and therefore a lower infection rate might be expected. We also had one particularly troublesome case where the patient did get repeated infections after coronectomy, and the decision was made to surgically remove the retained roots, which were found to be perforated by the inferior alveolar nerve. Despite removing the tooth fragments as atraumatically as possible, this patient did suffer inferior alveolar nerve involvement, which after 6 months has largely resolved, but not completely. The patient still has about a 10% nerve involvement, fortunately manifest as paresthesia and not dysesthesia. Using our technique of lingual nerve retraction, we have had a transient lingual paresthesia rate of slightly above 1% (eight cases), all but one of which resolved over 10 days. This last case did resolve completely but took 5 months to do so, which was concerning. Presumably these injuries are stretch injuries of the lingual nerve. We have no other cases of inferior alveolar nerve involvement.

ALTERNATIVE TECHNIQUES

Since publications commenced on coronectomy, a small number of alternative techniques have been advocated to avoid inferior alveolar nerve damage when removing lower third molars that appear to be intimately related to the nerve.

Orthodontic Extrusion of the Third Molars

Bonetti and others have published on the technique whereby an orthodontic bracket is attached to the impacted third molar, orthodontic traction applied, and the tooth pulled away from the inferior alveolar nerve and subsequently removed without nerve involvement.[44–46] Again, presumably if the roots are directly perforated by the nerve, it would not be possible to extrude the tooth without the nerve being affected. This

technique is obviously time consuming (and presumably costly) but may be indicated in certain circumstances.

Sequential Removal of Small Portions of the Occlusal Surface of the Impacted Third Molar

The technique of sequential removal of small portions of the occlusal surface of the impacted third molar such that it can erupt further until it moves far enough away from the nerve so that it can be safely removed was advocated by Tolstunov and coworkers,[47] under the name of pericoronal ostectomy. Presumably one does need adequate access to the crown of the tooth to remove 1 or 2 mm of the occlusal surface and whichever surface is causing the impaction at the time, and again if the tooth is actually perforated by the nerve, presumably it will not erupt.

SUMMARY

Coronectomy (also called intentional root retention or partial odontectomy) should be considered in cases of patients older than 25, where there appears to be an intimate relationship (low, medium, or high risk) between the roots of a retained lower third molar (or occasionally second or even first molars) and the inferior alveolar nerve, in circumstances where it is not contraindicated. It may be used on younger patients with a medium to high risk of inferior alveolar nerve damage. The decision to use this technique is currently made with the aid of CBCT scans. The short- to medium-term success rate seems to be excellent, but long-term studies are not yet available and could influence the conclusions.

REFERENCES

1. O'Riordan BC. Uneasy lies the head that wears the crown. Br J Oral Maxillofac Surg 1997;35:209.
2. Pogrel MA, Lee JS, Muff DF. Coronectomy: a technique to protect the inferior alveolar nerve. J Oral Maxillofac Surg 2004;62:1447.
3. Drage NA, Renton T. Inferior alveolar nerve injury related to mandibular third molar surgery: an unusual case presentation. Oral Surg Oral Med Oral Pathol Oral Radiol Endod 2002;93:358.
4. Freedman GL. Intentional partial odontectomy: review of cases. J Oral Maxillofac Surg 1997; 55:524.
5. Alantar A, Roisin-Chausson MH, Commissionat Y, et al. Retention of third molar roots to prevent damage to the inferior alveolar nerve. Oral Surg Oral Med Oral Pathol Oral Radiol Endod 1995; 80:126.

6. Zola MB. Avoiding anesthesia by root retention. J Oral Maxillofac Surg 1993;51:954.

7. Freedman GL. Intentional partial odontectomy: report of case. J Oral Maxillofac Surg 1992;50:419.

8. Knutsson K, Lysell L, Rohlin M. Postoperative status after partial removal of the mandibular third molar. Swed Dent J 1989;13:15.

9. Howe GL, Poynton HG. Prevention of damage to the inferior alveolar nerve during the extraction of mandibular third molars. Br Dent J 1960;109:355.

10. Blaeser BF, August MA, Donoff RB, et al. Panoramic radiographic risk factors for inferior alveolar nerve injury after third molar extraction. J Oral Maxillofac Surg 2003;61:417.

11. Rood JP, Shehab BA. The radiological prediction of inferior alveolar nerve injury during third molar surgery. Br J Oral Maxillofac Surg 1990;28:20.

12. Nakagawa Y, Ishii H, Nomura Y, et al. Third molar position: reliability of panoramic radiography. J Oral Maxillofac Surg 2007;65:1303.

13. Matzen LH, Christensen J, Hintze H, et al. Influence of cone beam CT on treatment plan before surgical intervention of mandibular third molars and impact of radiographic factors on deciding on coronectomy vs surgical removal. Dentomaxillofac Radiol 2013; 42:98870341.

14. Cilasun U, Yildirim T, Guzeldemir E, et al. Coronectomy in patients with high risk of inferior alveolar nerve injury diagnosed by computed tomography. J Oral Maxillofac Surg 2011;69:1557.

15. Hatano Y, Kurita K, Kuroiwa Y, et al. Clinical evaluations of coronectomy (intentional partial odontectomy) for mandibular third molars using dental computed tomography: a case-control study. J Oral Maxillofac Surg 2009;67:1806–14.

16. Tantanapornkul W, Okouchi K, Fujiwara Y, et al. A comparative study of cone-beam computed tomography and conventional panoramic radiography in assessing the topographic relationship between the mandibular canal and impacted third molars. Oral Surg Oral Med Oral Pathol Oral Radiol Endod 2007;103:253.

17. Susarla SM, Dodson TB. Preoperative computed tomography imaging in the management of impacted mandibular third molars. J Oral Maxillofac Surg 2007;65:83.

18. Dodson TB. Role of computerized tomography in management of impacted mandibular third molars. N Y State Dent J 2005;71:32.

19. Ohman A, Kivijarvi K, Blomback U, et al. Pre-operative radiographic evaluation of lower third molars with computed tomography. Dentomaxillofac Radiol 2006;35:30.

20. Chalmers E, Goodall C, Gardner A. Coronectomy for infraoccluded lower first permanent molars: a report of two cases. J Orthod 2012;39:117.

21. Renton T. Notes on coronectomy. Br Dent J 2012; 212:323.

22. Patel V, Sproat C, Samani M, et al. Unerupted teeth associated with dentigerous cysts and treated with coronectomy: mini case series. Br J Oral Maxillofac Surg 2013;51:644.

23. Sencimen M, Ortakoglu K, Aydin C, et al. Is endodontic treatment necessary during coronectomy procedure? J Oral Maxillofac Surg 2010; 68:2385.

24. Patel V, Sproat C, Kwok J, et al. Histological evaluation of mandibular third molar roots retrieved after coronectomy. Br J Oral Maxillofac Surg 2014;52: 415–9.

25. Leung YY, Cheung LK. Coronectomy of the lower third molar is safe within the first 3 years. J Oral Maxillofac Surg 2012;70:1515.

26. Zola M. Re: M. Sencimen, et al: Is endodontic treatment necessary during coronectomy procedure? J Oral Maxillofac Surg 68, 2010. J Oral Maxillofac Surg 2011;69:1269 [author reply: 1269].

27. Zallen RD, Massoth NA. Antibiotic usage for coronectomy: is it necessary? J Oral Maxillofac Surg 2005;63:572 [author reply: 572].

28. Pogrel MA. Coronectomy to prevent damage to the inferior alveolar nerve. Alpha Omegan 2009;102:61.

29. Johnson DI, Kelly JF, Flinton RJ, et al. Histologic evaluation of vital root retention. J Oral Surg 1974; 32:829.

30. Plata RL, Kelln EE, Linda L. Intentional retention of vital submerged roots in dogs. Oral Surg Oral Med Oral Pathol 1976;42:100.

31. Whitaker DD, Shankle RJ. A study of the histologic reaction of submerged root segments. Oral Surg Oral Med Oral Pathol 1974;37:919.

32. Patel V, Gleeson CF, Kwok J, et al. Coronectomy practice. Paper 2: complications and long term management. Br J Oral Maxillofac Surg 2013;51:347.

33. Renton T, Hankins M, Sproate C, et al. A randomised controlled clinical trial to compare the incidence of injury to the inferior alveolar nerve as a result of coronectomy and removal of mandibular third molars. Br J Oral Maxillofac Surg 2005;43:7.

34. Leung YY, Cheung LK. Safety of coronectomy versus excision of wisdom teeth: a randomized controlled trial. Oral Surg Oral Med Oral Pathol Oral Radiol Endod 2009;108:821.

35. Dolanmaz D, Yildirim G, Isik K, et al. A preferable technique for protecting the inferior alveolar nerve: coronectomy. J Oral Maxillofac Surg 2009;67: 1234.

36. O'Riordan BC. Coronectomy (intentional partial odontectomy of lower third molars). Oral Surg Oral Med Oral Pathol Oral Radiol Endod 2004;98:274.

37. Monaco G, de Santis G, Gatto MR, et al. Coronectomy: a surgical option for impacted third molars in

close proximity to the inferior alveolar nerve. J Am Dent Assoc 2012;143:363.

38. Geisler S. Coronectomy is an effective strategy for treating impacted third molars in close proximity to the inferior alveolar nerve. J Am Dent Assoc 2013; 144:1172.

39. Long H, Zhou Y, Liao L, et al. Coronectomy vs. total removal for third molar extraction: a systematic review. J Dent Res 2012;91:659.

40. Pogrel MA. An update on coronectomy. J Oral Maxillofac Surg 2009;67:1782.

41. Leung YY, Cheung LK. Can coronectomy of wisdom teeth reduce the incidence of inferior dental nerve injury? Ann R Australas Coll Dent Surg 2008;19:50.

42. Leizerovitz M, Leizerovitz O. Modified and grafted coronectomy: a new technique and a case report with two-year followup. Case Rep Dent 2013;2013: 914173.

43. Goto S, Kurita K, Kuroiwa Y, et al. Clinical and dental computed tomographic evaluation 1 year after coronectomy. J Oral Maxillofac Surg 2012;70:1023.

44. Wang Y, He D, Yang C, et al. An easy way to apply orthodontic extraction for impacted lower third molar compressing to the inferior alveolar nerve. J Craniomaxillofac Surg 2012;40:234.

45. Bonetti GA, Parenti SI, Checchi L. Orthodontic extraction of mandibular third molar to avoid nerve injury and promote periodontal healing. J Clin Periodontol 2008;35:719.

46. Alessandri Bonetti G, Bendandi M, Laino L, et al. Orthodontic extraction: riskless extraction of impacted lower third molars close to the mandibular canal. J Oral Maxillofac Surg 2007;65:2580.

47. Tolstunov L, Javid B, Keyes L, et al. Pericoronal ostectomy: an alternative surgical technique for management of mandibular third molars in close proximity to the inferior alveolar nerve. J Oral Maxillofac Surg 1858;69:2011.

Current Concepts of Periapical Surgery

Stuart E. Lieblich, DMD[a,b,*]

KEYWORDS

- Periapical surgery • Endodontic surgery • Mineral trioxide aggregate (MTA) • Fractured tooth

KEY POINTS

- Preoperative decision-making is vital to determine potential success of periapical surgery.
- Adequate exposure of the root apical region is best approached via a sulcular-type incision.
- Surgical procedures include resection of 2 to 3 mm of the apical portion along with root end preparation and seal.
- The surgeon must decide if submission of periapical tissues to pathology is indicated.

PREOPERATIVE PLANNING

Although endodontic care is typically successful, in approximately 10% to 15% of the cases[1] symptoms can persist or spontaneously reoccur. It is known that many endodontic failures are due to the failure to place an adequate coronal seal. Therefore, there is the competing interest of observing the tooth following endodontic treatment to ascertain successful treatment versus placing a definitive restoration with an adequate coronal seal. Many endodontic failures will occur a year or more following the initial root canal treatment, often creating a situation wherein a definitive restoration has already been placed, creating a higher "value" for the tooth because it now may be supporting a fixed partial denture. A decision is then needed to determine if orthograde endodontic retreatment can be accomplished should periapical surgery be recommended or consideration of extraction of the tooth with loss of the overlying prosthesis.

Causes of endodontic failures can often be separated into biologic issues, such as a persistent infection, or technical factors, such as a broken instrument in the root canal system (**Fig. 1**), or transportation of the apex, perforation, and ledging of the canal. Failure of endodontic treatment is most commonly due to lack of an adequate coronal seal with the presence of bacteria within the root canal system and apical leakage. Continued infection may also result from debris displaced out the apex during the initial endodontic treatment. Technical factors alone are a less common indication for surgery comprising only 3% of the total cases referred for surgery,[2] yet it is this author's opinion that there is a higher success rate in these cases.

Before surgery, discussions with patients are critical in order for the patient to give appropriate informed consent. The particular risks of surgery based on the anatomic location (sinus involvement or proximity to the inferior alveolar nerve) need to be reviewed and documented. It is important to stress the exploratory nature of periapical surgery to the patient. Depending on the findings at surgery, a limited root resection with retrograde restoration may be placed. However, the patient and surgeon must also be prepared to treat fractures of the root or the entire tooth. Plans must be made preoperatively on how such situations will be handled should they be noted intraoperatively.

Surgical endodontics success rates have dramatically improved over the years with the developments of newer retrofilling materials and the

[a] Oral and Maxillofacial Surgery, University of Connecticut Health Center, Farmington, CT, USA; [b] Private Practice, Avon Oral and Maxillofacial Surgery, 34 Dale Road, Suite 105, Avon, CT 06001, USA
* Avon Oral and Maxillofacial Surgery, 34 Dale Road, Suite 105, Avon, CT 06001.
E-mail address: slieblich@avonomfs.com

Oral Maxillofacial Surg Clin N Am 27 (2015) 383–392
http://dx.doi.org/10.1016/j.coms.2015.04.009
1042-3699/15/$ – see front matter © 2015 Elsevier Inc. All rights reserved.

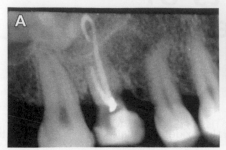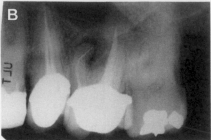

Fig. 1. Two examples of technical factors requiring apical surgery. Although less frequent in occurrence, the success rate is usually high because the canal system is likely well obturated. (*A*) Overfill of gutta percha causing symptoms including chronic sinusitis. (*B*) Broken endodontic instrument in apical third with pain and drainage.

use of the ultrasonic preparation. Previously cited success rates of 60% to 70% have now increased to more than 90% in many studies,[3,4] due to the routine use of ultrasonic retrograde preparation and the use of mineral trioxide aggregate (MTA [ProRoot MTA, Tulsa, Ok]) as a filling material. This significant improvement makes apical surgery a much more predictable and valuable adjunct in the treatment of symptomatic teeth. Most significantly, studies[5] show once the periapical bony defect is considered "healed" (reformation of the lamina dura or the case had healed by scar) the long-term prognosis is excellent. They reported 91.5% of healed cases still successful after a follow-up period of 5 to 7 years. Therefore, with adequate radiographic follow-up, the surgeon should be able to predict the long-term viability of the tooth and its usefulness to retain a prosthetic restoration.

There is some controversy in the endodontic literature that the use of magnification may improve outcomes in surgical management of endodontic failures. In a 2-part article by Setzer and colleagues,[6,7] a meta-analysis was reviewed on this subject of endodontic surgery. In part 1, they compared outcomes with traditional root end preparation with a rotary burr and amalgam filling versus more contemporary surgery with ultrasonic preparation and improved root end filling materials (Super-EBA, MTA). With the more contemporary surgery techniques, the outcomes improved from 59% to 94%. They then divided the literature into 2 groups in 2012: those using no magnification or loupes up to ×10 with those cases using the operating microscope or an endoscope with magnification greater than ×10. The group without magnification had a cumulative success rate of 88%, whereas the use of magnification had a pooled success rate of 93%. Of note was that no difference in success was noted for treatment of anterior teeth or premolars with or without magnification, but some improved success for molars (98% vs 90%).

The primary option for the treatment of symptomatic endodontically treated teeth is that of conventional retreatment versus the surgical approach. An algorithm for a decision regarding retreatment versus surgery versus extraction is presented in **Fig. 2**. In discussions with patients, the option of conventional retreatment should be discussed. Clinical studies though have not shown retreatment to be more successful than surgery and in fact one prospective study found surgical treatment to have a higher success rate.[8] Another study found a higher success rate with surgery from 2 to 4 years (77.8% vs 70.9%), but from 4 to 6 years it reversed to a success rate of 71.8% with surgery and 83% with conventional retreatment.[9] Although endodontic retreatment seems more "conservative," the removal of posts, reinstrumentation of the tooth, and removal of tooth structure increase the chance of fracture. Surgical treatment of failures also provides the opportunity to retrieve tissue for histologic examination to rule out a noninfectious cause of a lesion (**Fig. 3**).

The option of extraction with either immediate or delayed implant placement must also be discussed as an alternative to periapical surgery. There is no debate in dentistry that implants can outlast tooth-supported restorations. It is valuable therefore to have data to predict the expected success of the endodontic surgery so the patient can use that in their decision-making process. Factors that improve success are noted in **Table 1**. In cases of an expected poorer success rate, such as the presence of severe periodontal bone loss (especially the presence of furcation involvement), the decision to extract the tooth and place an implant may be a more efficacious and clinically predictable procedure.

There is a body of literature that supports the duration of restorations fabricated on endodontically treated teeth. Blomlof and Jansson[10] found surgically treated molars with healthy periodontal status had a 10-year survival rate of 89%, and Basten and colleagues[11] reported a 92% 12-yea

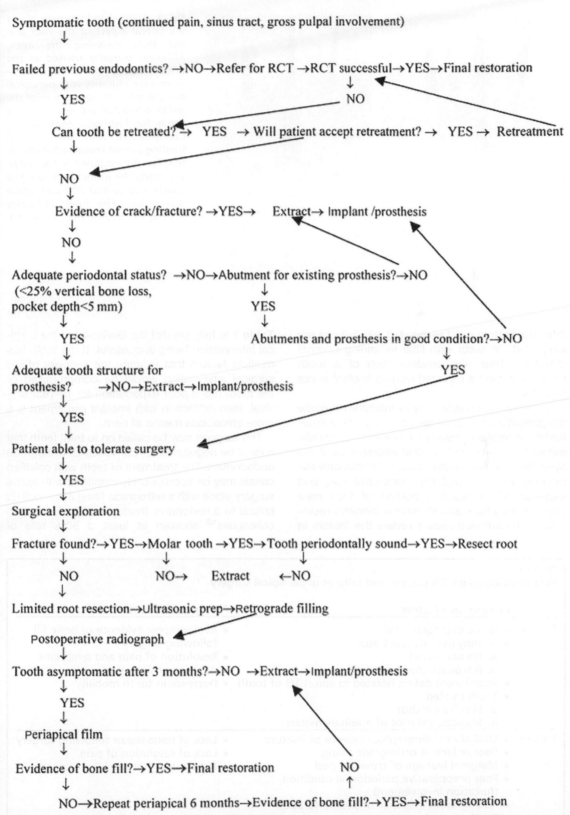

Symptomatic tooth (continued pain, sinus tract, gross pulpal involvement)
↓

Failed previous endodontics? →NO→Refer for RCT →RCT successful→YES→Final restoration
↓   ↓
YES   NO
↓

Can tooth be retreated? → YES → Will patient accept retreatment? → YES → Retreatment
↓

NO
↓

Evidence of crack/fracture? →YES→   Extract→ Implant /prosthesis
↓
NO
↓

Adequate periodontal status? →NO→Abutment for existing prosthesis?→NO
(<25% vertical bone loss,   ↓
pocket depth<5 mm)   YES
↓   ↓
YES   Abutments and prosthesis in good condition?→NO
↓   ↓
Adequate tooth structure for   YES
prosthesis?   →NO→Extract→Implant/prosthesis
↓
YES
↓

Patient able to tolerate surgery
↓
YES
↓
Surgical exploration
↓

Fracture found?→YES→Molar tooth →YES→Tooth periodontally sound→YES→Resect root
↓   ↓   ↓
NO   NO→   Extract   ←NO
↓
Limited root resection→Ultrasonic prep→Retrograde filling

  Postoperative radiograph
↓

Tooth asymptomatic after 3 months?→NO →Extract→Implant/prosthesis
↓
YES
↓
  Periapical film
↓

Evidence of bone fill?→YES→Final restoration   NO
↓   ↑
NO→Repeat periapical 6 months→Evidence of bone fill?→YES→Final restoration

Fig. 2. Algorithm for apical surgery. (*From* Lieblich SE. Periapical surgery: clinical decision making. Oral Maxillofac Clin North Am 2002;14:180; with permission.)

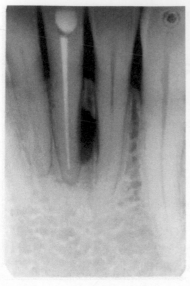 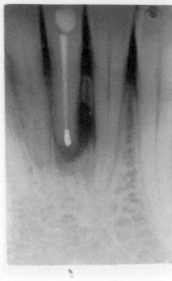

Fig. 3. Atypical radiolucency along the lateral aspect of the root and not truly involving the apex. Although correctly treated at the time of referral due to the nonresolving radiolucency with periapical surgery, the suspicious nature of the lesion warranted submission of the tissue for histologic examination. Confirmation with the original treating dentist revealed the indication for the endodontic treatment was solely the incidental finding of a radiolucency and vital pulp tissue was noted. The final pathology finding was a cystic ameloblastoma.

rate. The factors most associated with failures are long posts in teeth with little remaining coronal structure. Thus, the condemnation of a tooth because it can be replaced with an implant is not that clear.

An economic analysis may be indicated to guide the patient's decision. If the case has a final prosthetic restoration already in place, it is usually easier to recommend surgical intervention. If the symptoms do not resolve, the patient has only expended the additional time, operative risk, and expense of the surgical portion of their care because they have already have a definitive restoration. The surgeon should review the factors in

Table 1 to help predict the likelihood of the surgical intervention being successful. If the tooth has multiple factors that indicate the success of the surgical intervention would be compromised or the tooth has a poor expectation for 10-year survival, then extraction with implant placement is a more efficacious means of care.

The surgeon may be called on to treat teeth that cannot be negotiated for conventional orthograde endodontics. The treatment of teeth with calcified canals may be appropriately managed with apical surgery alone with a retrograde filling if the tooth is critical to a restorative treatment plan. Danin and colleagues[12] showed at least a 50% rate of

---

Table 1
Factors associated with success and failures in periapical surgery

	Preoperative Factors	Postoperative Factors

Success	• Dense orthograde fill
	• Healthy periodontal status
	  a. No dehiscence
	  b. Adequate crown:root ratio
	• Radiolucent defect isolated to apical 1/3 of tooth
	• Tooth treated
	  a. Maxillary incisor
	  b. Mesiobuccal root of maxillary molars
		• Radiographic evidence of bone fill following surgery
		• Resolution of pain and symptoms
		• Absence of sinus tract
		• Decrease in tooth mobility

Failure	• Clinical or radiographic evidence of fracture • Poor or lack of orthograde filling • Marginal leakage of crown or post • Poor preoperative periodontal condition (furcation involvement) • Radiographic evidence of postperforation • Tooth treated a. Mandibular incisor	• Lack of bone repair following surgery • Lack of resolution of pain • Fistula does not resolve or returns

complete radiographic healing and only one failure in 10 cases over a 1-year observation period in cases treated surgically only and without end-odontic treatment. Bacteria still remained in the canals of the tooth in 90% of these cases, which may lead to a later failure.

DETERMINATION OF "SUCCESS"

More complicated decisions are involved with teeth that have not been definitively restored. In that situation, not only does the surgeon have to consider the preoperative potential for the apical surgery to be successful but also often must determine when the case is deemed successful and the case can proceed to the final restoration. Once a final restoration is placed, considerably more time and expense have been invested and subsequent failure is more troublesome to the patient.

Rud and colleagues[13] retrospectively reviewed radiographs following apical surgery to determine radiographic signs of success. Their work showed that with a retrospective review of cases over at least 4 years after surgery, once radiographic evidence of bone fill occurs, noted as "successful" healing in their classification scheme, that tooth was stable throughout the remainder of their study period (up to 15 years). A waiting period of more than 4 years is not acceptable in contemporary practice, but their classification scheme has been validated over shorter observation times. They found that if radiographic evidence of bone fill of the surgical defect is noted, then the tooth remained a radiographic success over their observation periods. Many of the partially healing cases, noted as "incomplete healing" in their study, tended to move into the complete healing group during the 2 years following surgery, with very little changes throughout the next 4 years of observation.

An appropriate follow-up protocol is to obtain a repeat periapical film 3 months after surgery with critical comparison with the immediate postoperative film. If significant bone fill has occurred, mobility has decreased, pain is resolved, and no fistula is present, the case can proceed to the final restoration. However, if significant bone fill has not been noted, the patient should be recalled at 3 months for a new film. Rubinstein and Kim[14] found complete healing in 25.3% of cases in 3 months, and 34% took 6 months, 15.4% took 9 months, and 25.3% took 12 months. Small bony defects healed faster than large, which showed significant differences in their prospective study. In contrast, any increase in the size of the radiolucency or no improvement should caution the dentist about making a final restoration. If the situation is not clear at that time (6 months post-surgically), a temporary restoration, loaded for at least 3 months, is often a good "litmus test" of the success of the surgery and predictive as to whether the final restoration will last for some time.

THE CRACKED OR FRACTURED TOOTH

Preoperative radiographs and a careful clinical examination should be done with a high index of suspicion of a vertical root fracture (VRF) before undertaking surgery. Mandibular molars and maxillary premolars are the most frequent teeth to present with occult VRF. Although surgical exploration may be needed to definitively show the presence of a fracture (Fig. 4), subtle radiographic signs may alert the surgeon that a fracture is present, and the surgery is unlikely to be successful. Tamse and colleagues[15] looked at radiographs of maxillary premolars for comparison with the clinical findings at the time of surgery. Very few (1 of 15) teeth with an isolated, well-corticated periapical lesion had a VRF. In contrast, a "halo"-type radiolucency was almost always associated with a VRF (Fig. 5). This type of radiolucency is also known as a "J" type, wherein a widened periodontal ligament space connects with the periapical lesion, creating the "J" pattern.

It is critical in patient discussions to review the exploratory nature of the surgery; this author routinely uses that as a descriptor of the planned surgery. In cases of root fracture, a decision during surgery may need to be made to either resect a root or extract a tooth if a fractured root is found. Obtaining the appropriate preoperative consent as well as determining how the extracted tooth site will be managed (with or without a temporary removable partial denture) must be established before surgery commences.

CONCOMITANT PERIODONTAL PROCEDURES

The use of guided tissue regeneration, alloplastic or allogenic bone grafting, and root planing in conjunction with periapical surgery can be considered. In cases of severe bone dehiscence, the likelihood of success is known to be substantially compromised and may lead to the intraoperative decision to extract the tooth. Periodontal probing, before surgery, often will detect the presence of significant bony defects. Sometimes the amount of bone loss cannot be appreciated until the area is flapped (Fig. 6). Thus, the exploratory nature of the surgery needs to be stressed preoperatively with the patient.

The placement of an additional foreign body, such as a Gore-Tex (W.L. Gore and ASSOC,

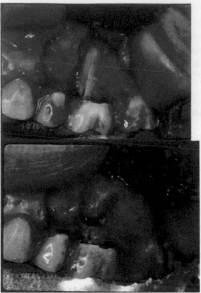

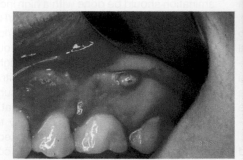

Fig. 4. VRF that was not diagnosed until explored at the time of surgery. The use of a sulcular flap permitted a resection of the mesiobuccal root and preservation of the tooth with its existing restoration.

Flagstaff, Ariz) membrane, to an area already infected is more likely to lead to failure of the surgery. Membrane stabilization and adequate mobilization of soft tissues to cover the membrane may increase the complexity of the surgical procedure. Nonresorbable membranes also require a second procedure for its removal that may not be tolerated by the patient as well as lead to an increase in scarring. A recent review by Tsesis and colleagues[16] seems to show a trend toward higher success with the use of resorbable membranes in cases of large defects and through and through lesions. However, this author does not advocate grafting or the use of membranes in conjunction with endodontic surgery. Clinical success defined as reduction in symptoms and spontaneous bone fill is routinely demonstrated without the use of allogenic bone or other GTR (guided tissue regeneration) procedures (**Fig. 7**).

SURGICAL PROCEDURES

Various steps are involved in the periapical surgical procedure. Initial exposure of the apical region is needed; this must allow access to the apex for the root resection. Approximately 2 to 3 mm of the root apex is resected. The root resection removes the end of the root containing the aberrant canals. Also, the further from the coronal portion of the tooth, the less dense the endodontic filling is likely to be.

Following the root resection, a thorough curettage of the periapical region is accomplished, being cognizant of local structures such as the maxillary sinus or the inferior alveolar nerve. Curettage removes periapical debris that may have been forced out the apex during the previous preparation of the root canal system. Tissue may be recovered at this time for histologic

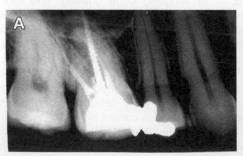

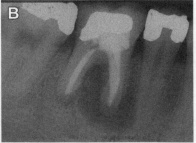

Fig. 5. (*A*) Example of a periapical lesion isolated to the apical one-third of the root. These lesions are rarely associated with a VRF. (*B*) In contrast, this type of radiographic lesion, known as a "halo" or "J" type of radiolucency, has ill-defined cortical borders and is most likely associated with a VRF.

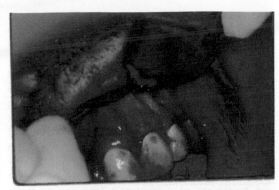

Fig. 6. A combination endodontic and periodontal lesion has a very low likelihood of success. The decision was made preoperatively to treat the tooth surgically because an adequate final restoration had already been placed. Otherwise, extraction with consideration of local bone grafting is indicated.

examination if indicated (see later discussion). A retrograde filling is then prepared with the use of the ultrasonic device; this creates a microapical restoration that is retentive due to the parallel walls. The ultrasonic device creates a very

conservative preparation and often finds unfilled canals or an isthmus of retained pulpal tissue connecting 2 canals, particularly in the mesiobuccal roots of maxillary first molars (**Fig. 8**). The ultrasonic preparation has been shown to be advantageous to the rotary drills because it will center the preparation along the long axis of the canal and significantly reduces the tendency to create root perforations.[17]

The retrograde filling is important to hermetically seal the root canal system, preventing further leakage of bacteria into the periapical tissues. Many filling materials have been used throughout the years and many do work well. The most contemporary material is MTA, which has been shown histologically to deposit bone around it. Its handling characteristics are somewhat different than other dental materials because it is hydrophilic and does not reach a full firm set for 2 to 4 hours; this is not clinically significant because the region is not load-bearing, at least for quite some time following the apical surgery. MTA has been shown to produce regeneration of cementum, something not seen with other root end filling materials.

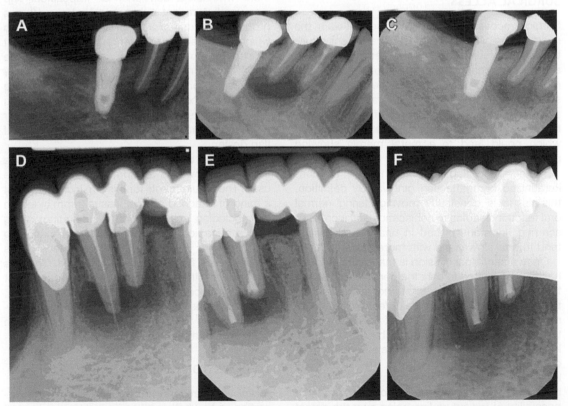

Fig. 7. (*A*) Large periapical lesion associated with teeth numbers 27 and 28 in proximity with an implant. Apical surgery was performed (*B*) with an MTA seal, and no graft or membrane was placed into the defect. (*C*) Bone fill after 3 months. (*D–F*) Similar situation with large defect successfully treated with apical surgery and MTA retrograde filling. No graft or membrane was placed in the defect.

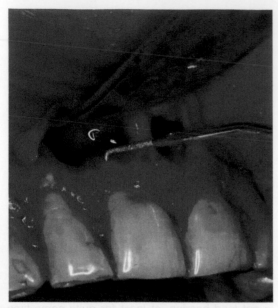

Fig. 8. The use of the ultrasonic tips allows a precise and retentive retrograde preparation. A minimal to no bevel is needed, which exposes less of the dentinal tubules in the apical aspect of the tooth.

SURGICAL ACCESS

Surgical access is a compromise between the need for visibility and the risk to adjacent structures. Many surgeons use the semilunar flap to access the periapical region. Although it provides rapid access to the apices of the teeth, it substantially limits the surgery to only a root resection and periapical seal. Proponents of this flap claim that it prevents recession around existing crowns, which could lead to a metal margin showing postoperatively.

The semilunar flap is placed entirely in the non-keratinized or unattached gingiva. By definition, this tissue is constantly moving during normal oral function, leading to dehiscence and increased scarring. Incisions placed in unattached tissues tend to heal slower and with more discomfort.

Once a semilunar incision is made, the surgeon has access limited to only the periapical region. If the root is noted to be fractured, extraction via this flap may lead to a severe defect. With a multi-rooted tooth, a root resection of one of the fractured roots may not be possible. In addition, localized root planing or other periodontal procedures cannot be accomplished. The size of the bone defect may be greater than that anticipated based on the preoperative radiographs and the possibility of the suture line being over the defect might cause the incision to open up and heal secondarily. Last, it is known that many cases of periapical surgery on maxillary molars and premolars will involve an opening into the sinus cavity.[18] The incision line with this type of flap might contribute to a postoperative oral-antral fistula.

In contrast, a sulcular incision with 1 or 2 vertical releases keeps the incision primarily within the attached gingiva, promoting rapid healing with less pain and scarring. Healing of the incision is facilitated by curetting the adjacent teeth and any exposed root surfaces before closure. The incision permits full observation of the root surface, leading to more accurate apical localization and treatment of a fractured root should it be discovered on flap reflection (see **Fig. 4**). By keeping the incision as far away from the sinus opening as possible and over healthy bone (vs a semi-lunar incision), the chance of an oral-antral communication is significantly reduced.

Concerns about sulcular incisions have revolved primarily around the concern for an esthetic defect that may be created with the shrinkage or loss of the interdental papilla. Jansson and colleauges[19] found the greatest predicator of papilla loss was the presence of a continued apical infection and no difference in the attachment whether a semilunar or trapezoidal flap was used. A recent publication by Velvart[20] has proposed the use of a "papilla-based incision" in which the triangle of interdental papilla is not incised and not mobilized during reflection of the flap. It reports maintenance of the papilla with little to no recession in contrast to mobilization of the papilla. Von Arx and colleagues[21] (**Fig. 9**) reviewed the papilla-based incision with the intrasulcular type and found less recession with this type of flap design.

In selected cases, an Ochsenbein and Luebke flap, also known as a submarginal flap, can be used. The requirements for this flap include at least a band of attached gingival tissue 2 mm in length (not including any periodontal pocketing) along with a periapical lesion that does not extend to this region.[22] Therefore, there are few cases whereby this flap design can be used. There is the limitation that if extraction of the tooth or root resection becomes the intraoperative decision, there becomes a technical complication. In addition, scarring is significant and recession can occur from that outcome.

TO BIOPSY OR NOT?

A clinical controversy has ensued over the consideration as to whether all periapical lesions treated surgically should have soft tissue removed and submitted for histologic evaluation. An editorial by Walton[23] questioning the rationale of submitting

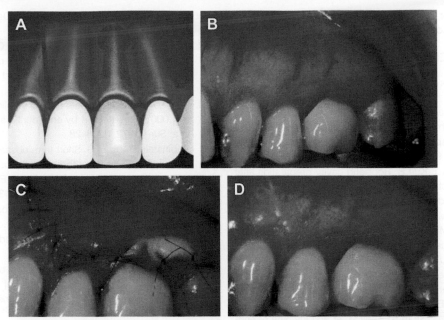

Fig. 9. Papilla-based incision has been shown to have less recession than the intrasulcular incision. (*A*) Schematic illustration of papilla based incision. (*B*) Baseline before apical surgery of the first molar. (*C*) Closure of incision. (*D*) One year follow-up picture. (*From* von Arx T, Vinzens-Majaniemi T, Bürgin W, et al. Changes of periodontal parameters following apical surgery: a prospective clinical study of three incision techniques. Int Endod J 2007;40(12):963; with permission.)

all soft tissue recovered for histologic examination ignited a series of letters to the editor. Organizations such as the American Association of Endodontists have stated in their standards that if soft tissue can be recovered from the apical surgery that it must be submitted for pathologic evaluation.

On cursory review, it seems that it is easier to make this recommendation than to have the surgeon determine if there is anything unusual about the case that warrants histologic examination. Walton[23] makes a convincing argument against the submission of all tissues, because similar-appearing radiolucencies that are not treated surgically do not have tissue retrieved for pathologic identification. It also is accepted that the differentiation between a periapical granuloma or periapical cyst has no direct bearing on clinical outcomes and therefore cannot be used as a rationalization for the submission of tissue.

The dilemma falls back to the surgeon that if a rare lesion should present itself in the context of a periapical lesion, and is not biopsied in a timely manner, the surgeon may have exposure in a potential malpractice suit. Many surgeons have a case or two in their careers that have "surprised" them based on the final pathologic diagnosis. However, careful review of these cases usually depicts a clinical situation inconsistent with a typical periapical infection (see **Fig. 3**).

An approach more logical than a purely defensive one is to set up guidelines on which it is determined submission of tissue was not indicated. These guidelines are listed in **Box 1**. It is recommended that the surgeon have documented in the record the rationale for electing not to submit tissue in each specific case. At a recent meeting of the American Association of Oral and Maxillofacial Surgeons, only 8% of those attending a symposium on endodontic surgery "always" submit

---

Box 1
Indications for nonsubmission of periapical soft tissues for histologic review

1. Clear evidence of pre-existing endodontic involvement of a tooth

   a. Pulpal necrosis was present, not just a periapical radiolucency

2. Unilocular radiolucency associated with apical one-third of the tooth

3. Lesion is not in association with an impacted tooth

4. No history of malignancy that could represent spread of a metastasis

5. Patient will return for follow-up examinations and radiographs

6. No tissue recovered at the time of surgery

tissue for histologic examination (Lieblich, personal communication, 2009).

REFERENCES

1. Kerekes K, Tronstad L. Long-term results of endodontic treatment performed with a standardized technique. J Endod 1979;5:83–90.

2. El-Siwah JM, Walker RT. Reasons for apicectomies. A retrospective study. Endod Dent Traumatol 1996;12:185–91.

3. Von Arx T, Kurl B. Root-end cavity preparation after apicoectomy using a new type of sonic and diamond-surfaced retrotip: a 1-year follow-up study. J Oral Maxillofac Surg 1999;57:656–61.

4. Zuolo ML, Ferreira MO, Gutmann JL. Prognosis in periapical surgery: a clinical prospective study. Int Endod J 2000;33(2):91–8.

5. Rubinstein RA, Kim S. Long-term follow-up of cases considered healed one year after apical microsurgery. J Endod 2002;28:378–83.

6. Setzer FC, Shah S, Kohli M, et al. Outcome of endodontic surgery: a meta-analysis of the literature—part 1: comparison of traditional root-end surgery and endodontic microsurgery. J Endod 2010;36:1757–65.

7. Setzer FC, Shah S, Kohli M, et al. Outcome of endodontic surgery: a meta-analysis of the literature—part 2: comparison of endodontic microsurgical techniques with and without the use of higher magnification. J Endod 2012;38:1–12.

8. Danin J, Stromberg T, Forsgren H, et al. Clinical management of nonhealing periradicular pathosis. Surgery versus endodontic retreatment. Oral Surg Oral Med Oral Pathol Oral Radiol Endod 1996;82(2):213–7.

9. Trobinejad M, Corr R, Handysides R, et al. Outcomes of nonsurgical retreatment and endodontic surgery: a systematic review. J Endod 2009;35(7):930–7.

10. Blomlof L, Jansson L. Prognosis and mortality of root-resected molars. Int J Periodontics Restorative Dent 1997;17:190–201.

11. Basten CH, Ammons WF, Persson R. Long-term evaluation of root-resected molars: a retrospective study. Int J Periodontics Restorative Dent 1996;16:206–9.

12. Danin J, Linder LE, Lundqvist G, et al. Outcomes of periradicular surgery in cases of apical pathosis and untreated canals. Oral Surg Oral Med Oral Pathol Oral Radiol Endod 1999;87(2):227–32.

13. Rud J, Andreasen JO, Jensen JE. A follow-up study of 1,000 cases treated by endodontic surgery. Int J Oral Surg 1972;1:215–28.

14. Rubinstein RA, Kim S. Short term observation of the results of endodontic surgery with the use of a surgical operation microscope and Super-EBA as root-end filling material. J Endod 1999;25:43–8.

15. Tamse A, Fuss Z, Lustig J, et al. Radiographic features of vertically fractured, endodontically treated maxillary premolars. Oral Surg Oral Med Oral Pathol Oral Radiol Endod 1999;88:348–52.

16. Tsesis I, Rosen E, Tamse A, et al. Effect of guided tissue regeneration on the outcome of endodontic treatment: a systematic review and meta-analysis. J Endod 2011;37(8):1039–45.

17. Wuchenich D, Meadows D, Torabinejad M. A comparison between two root end preparation techniques in human cadavers. J Endod 1994;20:279–82.

18. Feedman A, Horowitz I. Complications after apicoectomy in maxillary premolar and molar teeth. Int J Oral Maxillofac Surg 1999;28:192–4.

19. Jansson L, Sandstedt P, Laftman AC, et al. Relationship between apical and marginal healing in periradicular surgery. Oral Surg Oral Med Oral Pathol Oral Radiol Endod 1997;83:596–601.

20. Velvart P. Papilla base incision: a new approach to recession-free healing of the interdental papilla after endodontic surgery. Int Endod J 2002;35:453–60.

21. Von Arx T, Vinzens-Majanemi T, Jensen S. Changes of periodontal parameters following apical surgery. Int Endod J 2007;40:959–69.

22. Velvert P, Peters CI. Soft tissue management in endodontic surgery. J Endod 2005;31(1):4–16.

23. Walton RE. Routine histopathologic examination of endodontic periradicular surgical specimens—is it warranted? Oral Surg Oral Med Oral Pathol Oral Radiol Endod 1998;86(5):505.

Best Practices for Management of Pain, Swelling, Nausea, and Vomiting in Dentoalveolar Surgery

Stephanie J. Drew, DMD[a,b,c]

KEYWORDS

- Pain • Wisdom teeth • Nausea • Vomiting • Swelling • Outpatient

KEY POINTS

- Develop techniques to customize the outpatient experience and minimize these potential side effects.
- Review current therapies to minimize swelling, pain, and postoperative nausea and vomiting.
- Staying abreast of the current surgical and pharmacologic and even homeopathic methods of treating our patients' needs will ensure a safe outcome and good experience for our patients.

BEST PRACTICES FOR CONTROLLING PAIN, SWELLING, NAUSEA, AND VOMITING FROM DENTOALVEOLAR SURGERY

Currently, therapy for the management of patient comfort after third molar surgery should be directed toward procedure-specific pharmacologic techniques that will minimize the inflammatory and noxious stimulus to the soft and hard tissues of patients. The buzzword today is all about preemptive methods to minimize the untoward effects of the surgery and anesthesia.

Although good surgical technique is a given, all surgery creates injury to the soft and hard tissues when it is related to the removal of impacted teeth. Multiple biochemical cascades are activated on the first incision in the mucosa. End fibers of afferent neurons send signals created by the noxious stimulus to both the cerebral cortex and limbic system. The clotting cascade is also activated, bringing in not only the necessary clotting factors but also the next level of factors related to mounting an inflammatory response.

The inflammatory response to injury is the key to the development of pain and eventually swelling after any surgery. The inflammatory chemicals released from injury to tissue include prostaglandins, leukotrienes, bradykinin, and platelet-activating factors, to name a few. These chemicals, in turn, cause several chain reactions leading to vascular dilation and increased permeability, causing edema through interstitial fluid accumulation and increased tissue pressure.

The emotional response to pain and the actual surgical event can upregulate the response to the painful stimulus as well as the inflammatory stimulus that creates nausea, possibly leading to vomiting via the vagal pathways, our fight-or-flight mechanism.

Patient-specific factors to consider are their general health, including the possibility of a patient in chronic pain already on pain medications, drug

[a] Hofstra Medical school, 500 Hofstra University, Hempstead, NY 11549, USA; [b] University Hospital Stony Brook, 101 Nicolls Rd, Stony Brook, NY 11794, USA; [c] The New York Center for Orthognathic and Maxillofacial Surgery, 474 Montauk Highway, West Islip, NY 11795, USA
E-mail address: drdrew@nycoms.com

Oral Maxillofacial Surg Clin N Am 27 (2015) 393–404
http://dx.doi.org/10.1016/j.coms.2015.04.011
1042-3699/15/$ – see front matter © 2015 Elsevier Inc. All rights reserved.

abusers, immune compromise, and multiple allergies to medications. These patient issues are often difficult to manage well. Any patient that must take daily medication for any condition will need to be assessed for possible interactions between medications you would like to use, the surgical procedure needing to be done, and the risks of taking them off any medications they are using for their other health issues if indicated by the nature of the procedure.

Thus, there are multiple pathways that pharmacologic intervention can obtund, block, redirect, upregulate, or downregulate signals to improve the patients' physiologic experience as well as emotional experience postoperatively. Preventive measures should be considered in this light to decrease the pain, nausea, vomiting, and swelling associated with third molar surgery.

SURGICAL TECHNIQUE FROM OPENING TO CLOSING

The more difficult the surgery, the more likely the patient will experience pain, swelling and trismus after the surgical removal of third molars. Overall this impacts on the patient experience and quality of life for several days after the event. The grade of extraction thus correlates positively with the trauma created to remove a third molar. Parant grade I tooth is equivalent to a simple forceps removal, whereas grade IV will require bone cutting and flap reflection.[1] Understanding this relationship should guide the practitioner to provide appropriate surgical techniques to minimize trauma as much as possible. It also allows the surgeon to formulate a pharmacologic action plan for minimizing pain, swelling, and trismus after surgery.

If a tooth is impacted and requires removal, the thought of flap design and type of closure will play a role in minimizing pain, swelling, and trismus. Borgonovo and colleagues[2] recently evaluated the use of 3 different types of flaps in third molar surgery on postoperative discomfort. They described the use of an envelope flap, a triangular flap, or a trapezoidal flap. An envelope flap was the least traumatic with dissection; the trapezoidal flap required the most dissection, periosteal stripping, and perhaps manipulation or injury of the masseter muscle. An envelope flap led to the least amount of pain, trismus, and swelling.

Closure of the flaps created to remove third molars has also been evaluated in regard to preventing pain, swelling, and trismus.[3] Closure either primarily or secondarily did not seem to impact pain or facial swelling according to the reviews in these papers. However, secondary closure has been found to create less trismus. The use of primary closure versus a wound dressing was also assessed.[4] They found the use of a whitehead varnish dressing was more effective than primary closure to reduce swelling and trismus. Pain control was not changed with either method in this study. Logically the conclusion relates back to the initial issues described of tissue dissection and pain. The more dissection of either soft tissue or bone you do, the more it will create inflammation and, thus, increase pain.

PAIN CONTROL

As stated previously, the best method to control postoperative pain will be to minimize the soft and hard tissue trauma from surgery. However, this unfortunately cannot always be avoided in the removal of third molars. Pain control, thus, begins with good surgical technique. The rest is up to the medications we choose to use for our patients to interfere with the propagation of pain and the perception of pain. Of course, during the removal of third molars the surgeon will use a local anesthetic to achieve pain control for the short-term. Local anesthetics block the afferent neural stimuli from the surgery by blocking the low voltage–gated sodium channels on the cell membranes and, thus, interfere with the afferent signal propagation. Blocking of the afferent neural stimuli by the local anesthesia will reduce the hyperalgesia and allodynia associated with surgery. Block injections or infiltration of local anesthesia, long-acting or short-acting drugs, and postoperative use of extended-release local aesthetics should be considered. The block injections will last longer than the infiltration of medications regardless of the type of local used. The need for rescue injections, which further traumatize soft tissues and create more inflammation, should be reduced.

Many different types of local anesthetics are available for use in third molar surgery. Of interest is the speed of onset of the medication and how long it will last when it comes to postoperative pain management. Lidocaine is the standard that all other medications are compared. Recent studies of local anesthesia comparing the efficiency of lidocaine with articaine and bupivacaine have been published.[5–8] In all the onset of action of these drugs is not as much an issue in relation to postoperative pain as the duration of action. Bupivacaine should be the local anesthetic of choice when it comes to achieving long-acting postoperative anesthesia. Its duration of action has been reported to be as long as 10 hours. This duration is important because the initial onset of the maximum severity of postoperative pain peaks within the first several hours after surgery. This feature of bupivacaine will allow patients to get other medications on board that will be necessary to help decrease and control the swelling and pain of third molar removal before the onset of pain. Improvement of the patients' experience over all and quality of life after third molar surgical intervention may be the most important aspect of practice management.

On the forefront is the development of a delivery system for the extended release of bupivacaine. The Food and Drug Administration (FDA) has approved its use in 2011 for patients older than 18 years. The system has biodegradable and biocompatible lipid-based particles that contain the drug and allow diffusion over an extended time, which gives sustained local analgesia. The pharmaceutical company claims that the formulation should last up to 72 hours. This medication has been used in orthopedic surgery and soft tissue incisions of plastic and general surgery. There have been no publications in dentistry thus far, perhaps because of the cost of a single-dose vial being approximately $250. The development of pain, trismus, and swelling lasts for several days after the removal of third molars. Perhaps studies on the use of this medication delivery modality with sustained release should be considered.[9,10]

NONSTEROIDAL ANTIINFLAMMATORY DRUGS AND POSTOPERATIVE PAIN CONTROL

Prostaglandins are the primary mediator of acute postsurgical inflammatory changes and, thus, the development of pain. Inhibition of cyclooxygenase (COX) will prevent the production of prostaglandins. Two forms of COX exist: COX-1 and COX-2. It is known that COX-2 is primarily responsible for the cause of inflammation, pain, and fever. Nonsteroidal antiinflammatory drugs (NSAIDs) are drugs with antiinflammatory properties that work by blocking cyclooxygenase via the arachidonic acid pathway.

When these drugs are given preemptively before the initiation of surgical trauma, they are found to significantly reduce postoperative swelling, pain, and trismus.[11] One study compared the preoperative administration of oral diclofenac potassium, etodolac, and naproxen sodium on postoperative pain, swelling, and trismus.[12] The study concluded that diclofenac potassium was best at reducing swelling and equal to naproxen sodium and etodolac in reduction of pain and trismus. In another study, dexketoprofen trometamol was used in an intravenous preparation preoperatively and was found to have an excellent preemptive decrease in pain and swelling caused by third molar surgery.[13,14] The need for the use of postoperative

narcotic medications for breakthrough pain is better controlled with the preemptive use of NSAIDs.

Gastrointestinal (GI) complications, including upset and hemorrhage, have been known side effects of NSAID medications. Those drugs developed to be selective COX-2 inhibitors have less risk for damage to the GI mucosa.[15] Selective COX-2 inhibitor drugs, such as loxoprofen sodium and celecoxib, have been recently compared and found to be clinically compatible in the management of decreasing pain after third molar extraction.[16]

NARCOTICS

Hydrocodone, oxycodone, and codeine have been the go-to narcotics for the control of postoperative pain resulting from dentoalveolar surgery. These drugs have a place in our armamentarium, but their use must be monitored for abuse potential. While they work well in changing the perception of pain and centrally mediating the response, their side effects may overrun the benefits of use. Nausea, vomiting, constipation, dizziness, and allergy should be monitored during their use. These drugs are usually delivered in combination with acetaminophen. The potential for toxic levels of the acetaminophen must also be monitored.[17] Often these drugs can be used in combination with an antiinflammatory drug, such as ibuprofen, to enhance the response to pain control.

Tramadol is a centrally acting opiate that also has the properties of inhibiting serotonin reuptake.[18–20]

ACETAMINOPHEN

This drug is a centrally acting analgesic and antipyretic. The analgesic effects of this drug are created by it acting centrally by raising the pain threshold through what is thought to be inhibition of the nitric oxide pathway mediated by a variety of neurotransmitters, including N- methyl-D-aspartate and substance P. Although acetaminophen is one of the oldest and most widely prescribed analgesic drugs, its analgesic efficiency has been found to be improved by combining it with NSAID medications, such as ibuprofen.[21–24] These new combination medications or just combining them on your own may obviate or decrease the need for narcotic use in many patients.

Toxic levels of acetaminophen, especially affecting the liver, can increase quickly if the medication is not used appropriately, especially in the pediatric population. Recently, the FDA decreased the maximum daily dose of N-Acetyl-p-Aminophenol (APAP) from 4 g/d to 3 g/d because of the prevalence of hepatic injury. The FDA has also stated that single doses greater than 325 mg may cause liver toxicity (FDA 2014 http://www.fda.gov/drugs/drugsafety/safeuseinitiative/ucm230396.htm).

PSYCHOLOGY OF PAIN

Anxiety and fear can upregulate the pain signals received in the limbic system to create a hyper response to a painful stimulus. This center in the brain is responsible for the emotional component to our perception of a painful stimulus. The afferent fibers cross over from the trigeminal nucleus. As they do, they send off signals to this area as well as to the sensory cortex. There is neurochemical stimulation of the pathways that bring about the fear and anxiety known to be created from painful experiences.[25] This protective mechanism is a way that the signals are upregulated to enhance the emotional response and, thus, increase the reaction and response to a painful stimulus, not in proportion with the actual injury. In reality, this is a signal to get away from the noxious stimulus that is threatening our well-being.

SWELLING

Inflammation is the local physiologic response to tissue injury. The early stage of inflammation has fibrin and neutrophil polymorphs accumulation in the extracellular space of the damaged tissues. Three processes occur during this time: The vessels change in diameter; vascular permeability is changed and fluid exudate forms; and the cellular exudates of neutrophil polymorphs emigrate into the extravascular space. The chemical mediators of acute inflammation include histamine, prostaglandins, leukotrienes, serotonin, and various cytokines.

The prevention of inflammation and, thus, swelling is the goal of reducing postoperative pain and decreased quality of life after third molar surgery. Inflammatory mediator's processes can last up to 96 hours. Of note are the multiple steps along the biochemical pathways to inflammation and then swelling and pain that can be blocked with medications to prevent and decrease this postsurgical phenomenon.

STEROIDS

Corticosteroids have been the most common medications used to treat and prevent swelling and edema after surgery. They are immunosuppressive agents blocking both the early and late stages of inflammation. By inhibiting phospholipase A2, the release of arachidonic acid will be reduced at the site of inflammation. This reduction will decrease the synthesis of prostaglandins and leukotrienes and the accumulation of neutrophils.

In other words, steroids decrease swelling and, thus, pain by decreasing the action of pain mediators.

The delivery of steroids to patients can be via oral, intramuscular injection, or intravenous methods. One recent study compared the different routes of administration of methylprednisolone on edema and trismus after third molar surgery.[26] They found that the systemic application of a steroid was more effective on increasing range of motion. However, the direct injection of the steroid into the musculature had the best effect on decreasing postoperative swelling. Another study by Ehsan and colleagues[27] looked at the effect of *preoperative* submucosal administration of dexamethasone injection on swelling and trismus. They found that this injection was very effective in reducing the postoperative swelling and trismus associated with third molar removal. An update on the use of corticosteroids use in third molar surgery literature review revealed similar results. The administration of corticosteroids in the preoperative period via the parenteral route has the greatest impact on reducing postoperative swelling and trismus.[28]

Comparing corticosteroid administration versus NSAIDs for the relief of pain, swelling, and trismus has also been studied. The preemptive intravenous administration of tenoxicam (NSAID) was compared with the intravenous administration of methylprednisolone on pain, swelling, and trismus after wisdom teeth extraction.[29] Because the mechanism of action of these drugs has its effects on different parts of the inflammatory pathways, comparing the efficacy of them will be important in deciding which one to use. The oxicam group of NSAIDs works on the inhibition of cyclooxygenase and lipoxygenase enzymes. This action will prevent prostaglandin and leukotriene formation. Thus, it decreases the active oxygen radicals and inhibits migration and phagocytosis of leukocytes. This drug also has antipyretic, analgesic effects and also inhibits thrombocyte aggregation. Methylprednisolone inhibits macrophage development and decreases fibroblast formation and suppresses the immune system. It stabilizes cell membranes and reduces kinin and bradykinin formation and blocks histamine. The preemptive intravenous dosing of these drugs had both a positive and equal impact on postoperative control of pain and swelling. However, the use of methylprednisolone had better relief of trismus.

The comparison of preemptive administration of by-mouth prednisolone (steroid) to celecoxib (NSAID) on trismus and pain after third molar extractions was also studied. Once again, these drugs have different mechanisms of action. They found no difference in trismus; however, pain was better controlled with preemptive celecoxib.[30]

PROTEASE INHIBITORS

Complications of steroid use are well known. These complications include suppression of the immune system, hypertension, hyperglycemia, and suppression of adrenal corticosteroid activity. Alternative therapies for the use of steroids have been studied. Another class of drugs called *serine protease inhibitors* have been evaluated to compare their effectiveness in controlling pain and swelling after third molar surgery against the use of dexamethasone.[31] The drug aprotinin was used in this study delivered by submucosal injections before incision. This drug works by inhibiting the action of kallikrein and bradykinin. It also has a property to reduce bleeding. The dexamethasone was given intravenously 30 minutes before surgery. This study proved that aprotinin was better than dexamethasone in controlling postoperative swelling and pain after third molar surgery.

THE POWER OF THE PINEAPPLE

Bromelain is a proteolytic enzyme obtained from *Ananas comosus*, or pineapple plant. It is a potent antiinflammatory and antiedematous substance. The natural substance works by blocking bradykinin and its modulation of prostaglandin synthesis. Ordesi and colleagues[32] studied the effect of this plant enzyme on reducing postoperative pain and swelling after third molar surgery. Bromelain was found to significantly reduce the swelling and inflammation of third molar surgery. When taking bromelain tablets before surgery to 4 days after surgery compared with diclofenac sodium tablets started the day before surgery until 4 days after surgery, it was found to have compatible results on the effect of reducing pain and swelling and trismus after third molar removal.[33] This natural supplement may be considered as an alternative to NSAID therapy for improving the postoperative course.

LOW-LEVEL LASER ENERGY IRRADIATION

Low-level laser energy irradiation has been used locally at the surgical site in an attempt to decrease pain, swelling, and trismus after third molar removal while also increasing tissue healing. The laser treatment is typically given both intraorally and extraorally. The benefit of trismus reduction has been reported as well as decreasing pain and swelling. The decrease in pain with this technique comes from the reduction in edema, hemorrhage, and neutrophil infiltration and inflammatory cytokines and enzymes. The swelling is reduced by accelerating the regeneration of lymph vessels and decreasing vascular permeability.[34–37]

OTHER METHODS TO DECREASE SWELLING

Topical hyaluronic acid spray was recently introduced as a way to reduce swelling and trismus postoperatively. A recent study was done to compare it with the use of benzydamine. They were used as a spray: 2 pumps to the extraction sites 3 times a day for 7 days. It was found that the hyaluronic acid was more effective at reducing swelling and trismus. It had no effect on pain.[38] Further studies are needed.

Another recent study looked at the impact of warm saline rinses on the development of inflammation or osteitis postoperatively. They concluded that the rinses helped prevent the osteitis; however, the normal inflammatory response from surgical trauma is unavoidable and will not be prevented by the rinses.[39]

POSTOPERATIVE NAUSEA AND VOMITING

Nausea and vomiting are two of the most undesirable causes of patient dissatisfaction after third molar removal. Postoperative nausea and vomiting (PONV) after oral surgery can arise from multiple causes and lead to a myriad of complications, including dehydration and wound dehiscence and, in the worst case scenario, aspiration during the postoperative period. Controlling the potential causes of this complication may benefit patients and improve the overall experience by avoiding this issue when possible. Understanding the potential causes of PONV enables surgeons to see how to possibly modify their patients' behavior and make pharmacologic choices for maximum benefit.

There are 3 areas to address: the patients' risk factors, the anesthetic choices, and the type of surgery done. Adequate management of PONV should include an evaluation of the risk factors associated with developing nausea, creating a plan for the anesthetic drug choices, and possibly planning to use prophylactic premedication as well as a plan for rescue antiemetic medications.

There are 2 risk scoring systems available to help in patient risk assessment for PONV. In the adult patient population, the Apfel risk scoring system has been used (**Box 1**).[40] In the pediatric population, the Eberhart scale is used (**Box 2**). Risks factors associated with higher incidences of nausea and vomiting may include the types of anesthetic agents used, the length of surgery,

Box 1
Apfel score: for adult patients

Risk factors get one point each up to a total of 4 points

Risks assessed

　Female sex

　Nonsmoker

　History of motion sickness or PONV

　Use of opioids during surgery or after surgery

Interpretation of risk

　Score of 0 still have a 9% risk of PONV

　Score of 1 low risk has a 20% risk of PONV

　Score of 2 moderate risk has a 39% risk of PONV

　Score of 3 high risk has a 60% risk of PONV

　Score of 4 high risk has a 78% risk of PONV (especially when narcotics are used)

Adapted from Apfel CC, Laara E, Kiovuranta M, et al. A simplified risk score for predicting postoperative nausea and vomiting: conclusions from cross validations between two centers. Anesthesiology 1999;91:693–700.

Box 2
Eberhart score

Risk factors get one point up to a total of 4 points

Risks assessed

　Surgery ≥30 minutes

　Age ≥3 years old

　Strabismus surgery

　History of POV or PONV in relatives

Interpretation of risk

　Score of 0 has 10% risk of PONV

　Score of 1 has 10% risk of PONV

　Score of 2 has 30% risk of PONV

　Score of 3 has 55% risk of PONV

　Score of 4 has 70% risk of PONV

Adapted from Eberhart LH, Geldner G, Kranke P, et al. The development and validation of a risk score to predict the probability of postoperative vomiting in pediatric patients. Anesth Analg 2004;99(6):1630–7.

the site of surgery, patient sex, and postoperative use of opioids. In a recent poster presented at the American Association of Oral and Maxillofacial Surgeons 2014 annual meeting, Ashrafi and colleagues[41] presented their preliminary results on trying to identify risk factors specific to ambulatory anesthesia in the third molar surgery patient population. The incidence of nausea in the oral surgery populations was 54.0% and vomiting 11.49%. However, none of the risk factors mentioned in the research for the general anesthesia population were found to correlate with our ambulatory oral surgery population. One reason could be their small sample size. Nonetheless, these factors deserve further evaluation to see if there are any areas where we can control PONV or postdischarge nausea and vomiting (PDNV) with good anesthesia techniques and postoperative management of issues that are known to induce nausea and perhaps vomiting.

FEAR AS A CAUSE OF NAUSEA

Fight or flight with release of endogenous catecholamines and then with vagal stimulation may lead to nausea and perhaps syncope as well. This concept is simple but difficult to control unless you can create a relaxed environment in your offices and among yourself and staff. The patients' fears will only be enhanced in a chaotic setting. It is obvious that the fear factor can be managed pharmacologically in the beginning of sedation. However, emergence from anesthesia is also an important factor for these patients' overall experience. When a patient is extremely anxious, consideration to using a benzodiazepine during emergence may have a calming, although sedative effect. If a fearful patient wakes up feeling nauseated, it may induce fear and, thus, potentiate this unpleasant experience.

ANESTHETIC DRUGS AND NAUSEA

Side effects of multiple medications, especially narcotics and nitrous oxide, are thought to induce nausea in the postoperative period. Nitrous oxide works by releasing endogenous catecholamines. Ketamine also releases endogenous catecholamines. Opioid medications create nausea on many different levels. They delay gastric emptying, directly stimulate the chemoreceptor trigger zone, release serotonin, and increase the sensitivity of the vomiting reflex to signals from the vestibular apparatus. In a high-risk patient population, consideration may be given to modify the types of drugs used for sedation to avoid PONV. Total intravenous anesthesia with a combination of a short-acting narcotic and propofol has been studied and found to have less PONV compared with the use of volatile anesthesia in the general anesthesia patient population. This practice may be translated to the ambulatory setting such that our sedation techniques can also be modified to follow these protocols.[42]

LOCAL ANESTHESIA TOXICITY AND NAUSEA

Of special consideration is the careful monitoring of the amount of local anesthesia one uses in the setting of dental surgery. Toxic doses of local anesthetics may not only manifest with cardiac electrical changes but also nausea as an early sign of toxicity.

INGESTION OF BLOOD AND NAUSEA

The breakdown of blood into its various components and byproducts in the stomach may leave patients in a negative nitrogen balance situation and lead to the feeling of nausea. In the outpatient setting, adequate suturing, suctioning during surgery, special oval-shaped sponges that have been developed for throat screens during sedation, and perhaps using microfibrillar collagen plugs may be used to help obtain good hemostasis and minimize the amount of blood swallowed in the outpatient setting.

HYPOGLYCEMIA AND DEHYDRATION CAUSING NAUSEA

Patients who have not been eating or drinking before oral surgery either because of dental pain or observation of nothing-by-mouth status are all fluid depleted to some degree. Patients may also have a component of electrolyte imbalance, including hypoglycemia. These factors in combination with the potential fear-inducing experience may lead to the development of nausea both before and after surgery. Patients must be properly hydrated and have good postoperative pain control. This point is especially true for the patients who are operated on later in the day with sedation techniques. They may be observing nothing-by-mouth status longer than the first patient of the day.

SEX BIAS RELATED TO NAUSEA

Hormonal influences of the menstrual cycle create a propensity to have more nausea and vomiting within the first 8 days of menstruation. Several studies have noted this to increase the chances of vomiting by 4 fold.[43]

TYPE OF SURGERY

Hospital health care costs continue to increase. As a consequence, access to care in the hospital has been limited for many patients. This economic challenge has caused a shift in our choice of location to deliver care. Thus, more oral and maxillofacial procedures may be done in an ambulatory setting. The delivery of anesthesia, even in the ambulatory office setting, may need to be via general anesthesia with intubation using volatile anesthetics and/or total intravenous general anesthesia. From wisdom teeth to osteotomies to temporomandibular joint (TMJ) arthroscopy, the types of surgery are quite varied among the surgical population in the office setting today. The rule of thumb is the longer the procedure, the higher the risk of PONV. The longer the procedures, the more anesthesia is needed and the more clearance time is needed to get rid of the agents for anesthesia. All oral surgery procedures come with some inherent risks of swallowing blood. The more postoperative oozing, the higher the risks of PONV. Different anesthetic techniques in the ambulatory setting may be modified to minimize the risks of PONV by considering the patients' risks and timing of surgery when planning for determining either the anesthetic medications as well as the use of antiemetic drugs.

ANTIEMETIC MEDICATIONS FOR THE PREVENTION OF NAUSEA AND VOMITING: PREEMPTIVE VERSUS SYMPTOMATIC MANAGEMENT

Many different types of drugs may be used as an antiemetic (**Table 1**). These drugs include phenothiazines, butyrophenones, benzamines, anticholinergics, antihistamines, and serotonin receptor antagonists. Each drug type has a specific target and beneficial effect in preventing or alleviating PONV. Their individual side effects and potential drug interactions must be weighed against their benefits when considering their use either alone or in combination.

Phenothiazines (promethazine hydrochloride [Phenergan] and prochlorperazine [Compazine]) are direct dopamine-2 receptor antagonists. These receptors are located in the chemoreceptor trigger zone (CRTZ). They also have antihistaminic and anticholinergic effects. It is thought that these drugs can counter the emetic effects of opioids on the CRTZ. Benzamines (metoclopramide hydrochloride [Reglan] and trimethobenzamide hydrochloride [Tigan]) are also dopamine-2 antagonists. They work on both central and peripheral dopamine receptors. These medications also have serotonin or

Table 1
Quick reference guide for use of antiemetic drugs for PONV from oral and maxillofacial surgery procedures

Antiemetic Agent	Site of Action	Side Effects	Best Practice Uses	Trade Names
Phenothiazines	Dopamine-2 receptor antagonists in CRTZ antihistaminic Anticholinergic	Extrapyramidal Respiratory depression Sedation Hypotension Shorten local effects	Counter effects of opioids on CRTZ treating PONV Longer acting Lots of side effects Careful with patients with dystonia	Phenergan Compazine
Benzamines	Dopamine-2 receptor antagonist both central and peripheral	Serotonin receptor agonist/antagonist activity	Good for nausea caused by swallowing blood caused by increase gastric emptying	Reglan Tigan
Butyrophenones	Dopamine-2 receptor antagonist in CRTZ and area postrema α-blocker Anticholinergic	Arrhythmias: QT interval prolongation Hypotension Tachycardia	Use with caution in outpatient setting for PONV	Droperidol
Anticholinergics	Block acetylcholine action on the parasympathetic nervous system	Dry mouth Additive effects with opioids	Good for motion sickness and vertigo Consider in TMJ surgery or early ambulating patients See notes on pretreatment with scopolamine patch	Dramamine Scopolamine
Antihistamines	H-1 receptor inverse agonists with anticholinergic properties	Additive anticholinergic effects with opioids	Good for nausea caused by anxiety	Vistaril Atarax Cyclizine
Serotonin receptor antagonists	Block the CRTZ and peripheral vagal receptors liked to vomiting center	—	Fast onset Most expensive Has oral dissolving tablet (ODT) available Use to prevent or treat PONV	Zofran

5-hydroxytryptamine (5HT-3) receptor agonist/antagonist properties. The anticholinergics (dimenhydrinate [Dramamine] and scopolamine) block the action of acetylcholine on the parasympathetic nervous system. In the 2015 report by Brookes and colleagues[44] on using multimodal therapy to prevent PONV in patients with Le Fort I, they advocate for the use of preoperative transdermal scopolamine to alleviate the PONV associated with Le Fort surgery. Antihistamines (hydroxyzine [Vistaril], hydroxyzine hydrochloride [Atarax], and cyclizine) are H-1 receptor inverse agonists that have anticholinergic properties that work to prevent nausea. Serotonin 5HT-3 receptor antagonists (ondansetron hydrochloride [Zofran]) block in both the central nervous system at the CRTZ and peripheral receptors at the vagal terminals, which are linked centrally to the vomiting center.

The side effects of these drugs may cause anything from a dry mouth (anticholinergics), cardiac arrhythmia changes (butyrophenones), additive anticholinergic effects with opioids (anticholinergics and antihistamines), more sedation, hypotension, respiratory depression, extrapyramidal side effects and shortened desired effects of local anesthetics caused by increase epinephrine metabolism (phenothiazines), and headache, constipation, and dizziness (serotonin receptor antagonists).

Prophylactic use of antiemetic medications, such as ondansetron hydrochloride (Zofran), has been suggested as a way to prevent PONV.[45–47] These medications are serotonin receptor antagonists. One of the most challenging patients to manage postoperative nausea in is the tympanoplasty patient group. This patient population has been studied comparing the use of ondansetron versus dexamethasone versus placebo. They found using either the ondansetron or the dexamethasone was more effective in controlling PONV when compared with a placebo.[48]

However, the evidence to support prophylactic use of ondansetron on every patient is lacking in support in the oral and maxillofacial surgery literature because of the cost, safety, and adverse reactions reported when using these drugs. Several studies have compared the use of these medications against a placebo and have found equivocal results.[49–51] Thus, their routine prophylactic use cannot be advocated as an absolute at this time. A more logical approach would be to use the observation of more than one risk factor on the Apfel scale as well as type and predicted length of surgery and likelihood of swallowing a great deal of blood to guide the practitioner to consider using preemptive medications. Otherwise treat PONV symptomatically.[52,53]

Consideration to the use of anesthetic agents with antiemetic properties should also be considered (**Table 2**). The symptomatic treatment of PONV seems to be a more reasonable approach for these patients. Cruthirds and colleagues[54] have reviewed the pharmacology of the antiemetic drugs and the current therapies to prevent, manage, and treat PONV and PDNV. In this comprehensive paper they remind us that a 20% to 30% incidence of PONV and PDNV can be expected from sedation or general anesthesia in oral and maxillofacial surgery procedures. High-risk patients should be identified and treated prophylactically with antiemetic medications. The use of anesthetic medications with antiemetic properties should be considered if appropriate. The use of anesthetic medications with antiemetic properties should be considered if appropriate. The drugs one could consider may include Benzodiazepines, propofol, and dexamethasone. The addition of the steroid dexamethasone seems to decrease the likelihood of PONV. Minimize the use of opioids when appropriate, especially in the postoperative period. The same antiemetic medication should not necessarily be used again as rescue therapy if initial treatment of PONV fails. Silva and colleagues[55] called for development of protocols for preventing PONV in the orthognathic surgery population in 2006, and today Brookes and colleagues[44] have addressed these needs based on good science and understanding of multimodal approach to managing PONV in the orthognathic surgery population. Perhaps these protocols can be studied and modified for our outpatient surgical procedures in the future.

SUMMARY

Best practices refer to the most common and proven techniques used in medicine and dentistry that have predictable outcomes for our patients. Best practices are used as a guideline for the

Table 2
Commonly used anesthetic agents in oral and maxillofacial surgery and their effects

Anesthetic Agent	Emetic	Pain Control	Antiinflammatory	Anxiolytic
Lidocaine	+	+	—	—
Bupivacaine hydrochloride (Marcaine)	+	+	—	—
Mepivacaine hydrochloride (Carbocaine)	+	+	—	—
Articaine hydrochloride and epinephrine (Septocaine)	+	+	—	—
Midazolam	—	—	—	+
Diazepam (Valium)	—	—	—	+
Methohexital sodium (Brevital)	—	—	—	+
Fentanyl	+	+	—	+
Remifentanil	+	+	—	+
Ketamine	—	+	—	+
Propofol	—	+	—	+
Nitrous oxide	+	+	—	+
Volatile agents	+	+	—	+

surgeon to help in managing and preventing complications of surgery. The caveat is that not all patients will respond to our best practices protocols, but most do. Understanding the complex nature of the inflammatory response to our surgical trauma as well as the biochemical and then physiologic responses to the medications we use during surgery helps to also guide us in finding ways to decrease pain, swelling, nausea, and vomiting. Staying abreast of the current surgical, pharmacologic, and even homeopathic methods of treating our patient's needs will ensure a safe outcome and good experience for our patients.

REFERENCES

1. Pathak S, Vashisth S, Mishra S, et al. Grading of extraction and its relationship with post-operative pain and trismus, along with proposed grading for trismus. J Clin Diagn Res 2014;8(6):9–11.

2. Borgonovo AE, Giussani A, Grossi GB, et al. Evaluation of postoperative discomfort after impacted mandibular third molar surgery using three different types of flap. Quintessence Int 2014;45(4):319–30.

3. Carrasco-labra A, Brignardello-Petersen R, Yanine N, et al. Secondary versus primary closure techniques for the prevention of postoperative complications following removal of impacted mandibular third molars: a systematic review and meta-analysis of randomized controlled trials. J Oral Maxillofac Surg 2012;70(8):441–57.

4. Egbor P, Saheeb BD. A prospective randomized clinical study of the influence of primary closure or dressing on post-operative morbidity after mandibular third molar surgery. Niger J Surg 2014;20(2):59–63.

5. De Souza Am, Horliana AC, Simone JL, et al. Postoperative pain after bupivacaine supplementation in mandibular third molar surgery: splint-mouth randomized double blind controlled clinical trial. Oral Maxillofac Surg 2014;18(4):387–91.

6. Al-delayme RM. A comparison of two anesthesia methods for the surgical removal of maxillary third molars: PSA nerve block technique vs. local infiltration technique. J Clin Exp Dent 2014;6(1):e12–6.

7. Martinez-Rodriquez N, Barona-Dorado C, Martin-Ares M, et al. Evaluation of the anesthetic properties and tolerance of 1:100,000 articaine versus 1:100,000 lidocaine. A comparative study in surgery of the lower third molar. Med Oral Patol Oral Cir Bucal 2012;17(2):e345–51.

8. Sancho-Puchades M, Vilchez-perez MA, Valmaseda- Castellon E, et al. Bupivacaine 0.5% versus articaine 4% for the removal of lower third molars. A crossover randomized controlled trial. Med Oral Patol Oral Cir Bucal 2012;17(3):e462–8.

9. Portillo J, Kamar N, Melibary S, et al. Safety of liposome extended –release bupivacaine for postoperative pain control. Front Pharmacol 2014;5:1–6.

10. Saraghi M, Hersh EV. Three newly approved analgesics: an update. Anesth Prog 2013;60:178–87.

11. Zor ZF, Isik B, Cetiner S. Efficacy of preemptive lornoxicam on postoperative analgesia after surgical removal of mandibular third molars. Oral Surg Oral Med Oral Pathol Oral Radiol 2014;117(1):27–31.

12. Akbulut N, Ustuner E, Atakan C, et al. Comparison of the effect of naproxen, etodolac and diclofenac on postoperative sequels following third molar surgery: a randomized, double blind, crossover study. Med Oral Patol Oral Cir Bucal 2014;19(2):e149–56.

13. Cagiran E, Eyigor C, Sezer B, et al. Preemptive analgesic efficacy of dexketoprofen trometamol on impacted third molar surgery. Agri 2014;26(1):29–33.

14. Velasquez GC, Santa Cruz LA, Espinoza MA. Ketoprofen is more effective than diclofenac after oral surgery when used as a preemptive analgesic: a pilot study. J Oral Facial Pain Headache 2014;28(2):153–8.

15. Radhofer-Welte S, Rabasseda X. Lornoxicam, a new potent NSAID with an improved tolerability profile. Drugs Today (Barc) 2000;36(1):55–76.

16. Yamashita Y, Sano N, Shimohira D, et al. A parallel-group comparison study of celecoxib withloxoprofen sodium in thirs mandivular molar extraction patients. Int J Oral Maxillofac Surg 2014;43(12):1509–13.

17. Hawthorne J, Stein P, Aulisio M, et al. Opiate overdose in an adolescent after a dental procedure: a case report. Gen Dent 2011;59(2):e46–9.

18. Isiordia-Espinoza MA, Dejesus Pozos-Guillen A, Aragon-Martinez OH. Analgesic efficacy and safety of single dose tramadol and non-steroidal anti-inflammatory drugs in operations on the third molars: a systematic review and meta analysis. Br J Oral Maxillofac Surg 2014;52(9):775–83.

19. Gopalraju P, Lalitha RM, Prasad K, et al. Comparative study of intravenous tramadol versus ketorolac for preventing postoperative pain after third molar surgery—a prospective randomized study. J Craniomaxillofac Surg 2014;42(5):629–33.

20. Perez-Urizar J, Martinez-Rider R, Torres-Roque I, et al. Analgesic efficacy of lysine clonixinate plus tramadol versus tramadol in multiple doses following impacted third molar surgery. Int J Oral Maxillofac Surg 2014;43(3):348–54.

21. Qi DS, May LG, Zimmerman B, et al. A randomized, double-blind, placebo-controlled study of acetaminophen 1000mg versus acetaminophen 650mg for the treatment of postsurgical dental pain. Clin Ther 2012;34(12):2247–58.

22. Krasniak AE, Knopp GT, Svensson CK, et al. Pharmogenomix of acetaminophen in pediatric populations: a moving target. Front Genet 2014;5:314.

23. Moore PA, Hersh EV. Combining ibuprofen and acetaminophen for acute pain management after third-molar extractions: translating clinical research to dental practice. J Am Dent Assoc 2013;144(8): 898–908.

24. Balley E, Worthington HV, Coulthard P. Ibuprofen and/or paracetamol (acetaminophen) for pain relief after surgical removal of lower wisdom teeth. Cochrane database systematic review. Br Dent J 2014;216(8):451–5.

25. Torres-Lagares D, Recio-Lora C, Castillo-Dali G, et al. Influence of state anxiety and trait anxiety in postoperative in oral surgery. Med Oral Patol Oral Cir Bucal 2014;19(4):403–8.

26. Kocer G, Yuce E, Oncul AT, et al. Effect of the route of administration of methylprednisolone on oedema and trismus in impacted lower third molar surgery. Int J Oral Maxillofac Surg 2014;43:639–43.

27. Ehsan A, Ali Bukhari SG, Ashar, et al. Effects of preoperative submucosal dexamethasone injection on the postoperative swelling and trismus following surgical extraction of mandibular third molar. J Coll Physicians Surg Pak 2014;24(7):489–92.

28. Herrera-Briones FJ, Prados sanchez E, Reyes Botella C, et al. Update on the use of corticosteroids in third molar surgery: systematic review of the literature. Oral Surg Oral Med Oral Pathol Oral Radiol 2013;116(5):e342–51.

29. Ilhan O, Agacayak KS, Gulsun B, et al. A comparison of the effects of methylprednisolone and tenoxicam on pain, edema, and trismus after impacted lower third molar extraction. Med Sci Monit 2014;20:147–52.

30. Moghaddamina AA, Nosrati K, Mehdizadeh M, et al. A comparison study of the effect of prednisolone and celecoxib on MMO(maximum mouth opening) and pain following removal of impacted mandibular third molars. J Maxillofac Oral Surg 2013;12(2):184–7.

31. Akrakeri G, rai KK, Shivakumar HR, et al. A randomized clinical trial to compare the efficacy of submucosal aprotinin injection and intravenous dexamethasone in reducing pain and swelling after third molar surgery: a prospective study. J Maxillofac Oral Surg 2013;12(1):73–9.

32. Ordesi P, Pisoni L, Nannei P, et al. Therapeutic efficacy of bromelain in impacted third molar surgery: a randomized controlled clinical study. Quintessence Int 2014;45(8):679–84.

33. Majid OW, Al-Mashhadani BA. Perioperative bromelain reduces pain and swelling and improves quality of life measures after mandibular third molar surgery: a randomized, double-blind, placebo-controlled clinical trial. J Oral Maxillofac Surg 2014;72(6):1043–8.

34. Batinjan G, Zore Z, Celebic A, et al. Thermographic monitoring of wound healing and oral health-related quality of life in patients treated with laser (aPDT) after impacted mandibular third molar removal. Int J Oral Maxillofac Surg 2014;43:1503–8.

35. He WL, Yu FY, Li CJ, et al. A systematic review and meta-analysis on the efficacy of low-level laser therapy in the management of complication after mandibular third molar surgery. Lasers Med Sci 2014. [Epub ahead of print].

36. Sierra SO, deana AM, Ferrari RA, et al. Effect of low level laser therapy on the post surgical inflammatory process after third molar removal: study protocol for a double blind randomized controlled trial. Trials 2013;14:373.

37. Brignardello-Petersen R, Carrasco-lavara A, Arya I, et al. Is adjuvant laser therapy effective for preventing pain, swelling and trismus after surgical removal of impacted mandibular third molars? A systematic review and meta- analysis. J Oral Maxillofac Surg 2012;70(8):1789–801.

38. Koray M, Ofluoflu D, Onal EA, et al. Efficacy of hyaluronic acid spray on swelling, pain and trismus after surgical extraction of impacted mandibular third molars. Int J Oral Maxillofac Surg 2014;43(11): 1399–403.

39. Osunde OD, Adebola RA, Adeoye JB, et al. Comparative study of the effect of warm saline mouth rinse on complications after dental extractions. Int J Oral Maxillofac Surg 2014;43:649–53.

40. Apfel CC, Laara E, Kiovuranta M, et al. A simplified risk score for predicting postoperative nausea and vomiting: conclusions from cross validations tween two centers. Anesthesiology 1999;91:693–700.

41. Ashrafi A, Savoree S, Viswanath A. Post discharge nausea/vomiting after ambulatory anesthesia in oral surgery. Poster 04 AAOMS 2014. e-53.

42. Fujii Y, Uemura A, akano M. Small dose of propofol for preventing nausea and vomiting after third molar extraction. J Oral Maxillofac Surg 2002;60:1246–9.

43. Ramsay TM, McDonald PF, Faragher EB. The menstrual cycle and nausea or vomiting after wisdom teeth extraction. Can J Anaesth 1994;41(9): 798–801.

44. Brookes CD, Berry J, Rich J, et al. Multimodal protocol reduces postoperative nausea and vomiting in patients undergoing Le Fort I osteotomy. J Oral Maxillofac Surg 2015;73(2):324–32.

45. Talesh KT, Motamedi MH, Kahnamouii S. Comparison of ondansetron and metoclopramide antiemetic prophylaxis in maxillofacial surgery patients. Oral Surg Oral Med Oral Pathol Oral Radiol Endod 2011;111(3):275–7.

46. Rodrigo C, Campbell R, Chow J, et al. The effect of a 4-mg preoperative intravenous dose of ondansetron in preventing nausea and vomiting after maxillofacial surgery. J Oral Maxillofac Surg 1996;54(10): 1171–5.

47. Wagley C, Hackett C, Haug RH. The effect of preoperative ondansetron on the incidence of postoperative nausea and vomiting in patients undergoing outpatient dentoalveolar surgery and general anesthesia. J Oral Maxillofac Surg 1999; 57(10):1195–200.

48. Eidi M, Kolahdouzan K, Hosseinzadeh H, et al. A comparison of preoperative ondansetron and Dexamethasone in the prevention of post-tympanoplasty nausea and vomiting. Iran J Med Sci 2012;37(3):166–72.

49. Alexander M, Krishnan B, Yuvraj V. Prophylactic antiemetics in oral and maxillofacial surgery- a requiem? J Oral Maxillofac Surg 2009;67(9):1873–7.

50. Rodseth RN. Prophylactic antiemetics in oral and maxillofacial surgery- a requiem? –a response. J Oral Maxillofac Surg 2010;68(5):1212–3.

51. Alexander M. Prophylactic antiemetics in oral and maxillofacial surgery- a requiem?—Reply. J Oral Maxillofac Surg 2010;68(5):1213.

52. Beckley ML. Management of postoperative nausea and vomiting: the case for symptomatic treatment. J Oral Maxillofac Surg 2005;63(10):1528–30.

53. Kovac AL. The prophylactic treatment of postoperative nausea and vomiting in oral and maxillofacial surgery. J Oral Maxillofac Surg 2005;63(10):1531–5.

54. Cruthirds D, Simms PJ, Louis PJ. Review and recommendations for the prevention, management, and treatment of postoperative and post discharge nausea and vomiting. Oral Surg Oral Med Oral Pathol Oral Radiol 2013;115(5):601–11.

55. Silva AC, O'Ryan F, Poor DB. Postoperative nausea and vomiting (PONV) after orthognathic surgery: a retrospective study and literature reveiew. J Oral Maxillofac Surg 2006;64(9):1385–97.

Developing and Implementing a Culture of Safety in the Dentoalveolar Surgical Practice

James R. Hupp, DMD, MD, JD, MBA

KEYWORDS

• Culture of safety • Dentoalveolar practice • Risk management

KEY POINTS

- A culture of safety is the establishment and maintenance of organizational behavior in which members of the organization place a high priority on identifying and rectifying safety issues.
- Surgeons must take the lead in instituting a culture of safety and in continuing to nurture it over the long run; discussions of safety matters should be a standard agenda item for office meetings.
- The culture of safety in an oral-maxillofacial surgery dentoalveolar practice has several dimensions: (1) clinical care safety, (2) intraoffice guest and health care team safety, and (3) safety from extra-office dangers.

INTRODUCTION

Many industries face the problem of injuries due to accidents. Employee safety awareness programs are longstanding in manufacturing firms, where employees are exposed to dangerous environments. However, more recently, it has been recognized that patients too may suffer injuries while under the care of doctors. This finding has led to the culture of safety movement within the health care industry. This article reviews some of the background related to this relatively new focus on patient safety. The background is followed by a discussion of some practices hospitals have put in place to reduce the risk of patient injury. Then, the main thrust of this article focuses on how general concepts of a culture of safety can be applied to the oral-maxillofacial surgery (OMS) office, providing dentoalveolar surgical care.

THE CULTURE OF SAFETY CONCEPT

Although public safety has long been a focus of police and fire departments, government officials responsible for overseeing transportation, public spaces, and facilities, and elected officials creating regulations affecting food, drugs, and other matters, attention to safety in the health care industry is a relatively new development.[1] The works of Treadwell and colleagues[2] and Gawande,[3,4] among others, drew attention to the problem of patient safety in the US hospital industry. Their articles discuss how many foreseeable and preventable problems occur when patients require hospitalization. These injuries are due to wrong surgery site, improper drug administration, and infections caused by unexpected pathogens, among a host of other issues.[5] These errors were not complications of needed care; instead, the alarm was raised because of not recognizing them as safety issues.

The airline industry has a long history of a focus on safety.[6] This focus on safety arose because of the catastrophic results possible when a plane crashes. Once the hospital industry was sensitized to the common safety problems present in their organizations, many turned to safety practices used in the airline industry to address problems

School of Dental Medicine, East Carolina University, Greenville, NC, USA
E-mail address: jrhupp@me.com

Oral Maxillofacial Surg Clin N Am 27 (2015) 405–409
http://dx.doi.org/10.1016/j.coms.2015.04.008
1042-3699/15/$ – see front matter © 2015 Elsevier Inc. All rights reserved.

affecting hospital patients. The most important concept adopted by hospitals was the airline industry's culture of safety.

A culture of safety is the establishment and maintenance of organizational behavior in which members of the organization place a high priority on identifying and rectifying safety issues (**Box 1**). When hospitals work to develop a culture of safety, they strive to have all clinical staff members, including doctors, nurses, and medical technicians as well as others on the hospital staff who play a role in patient care, understand and accept the responsibility to identify and help to mitigate patient safety risks. Commonly, hospitals appoint safety officers to head the culture of safety activities. Such activities include establishing the use of checklists and operating room timeouts, blood bank storage and delivery protocols, handwashing routines, and drug administration algorithms. Institutions with an effective culture of safety establish safety monitoring and injury reporting protocols.[7,8] In addition, policies are designed to mandate root cause analysis of patient injuries, followed by meetings to develop and implement preventative practices that are then disseminated throughout the organization. As with any initiative of this magnitude, the institution's leadership plays a critical role in ensuring its success.

HOSPITAL SAFETY PRACTICES

Because most oral-maxillofacial surgeons work to some degree in hospitals, they are familiar with some of the practices hospitals now use to help protect patients from injuries. In the operating suite, most hospitals require surgeons to have patients initial the site of surgery before they begin the anesthesia process. Initialing the site of surgery has helped decrease the incidence of wrong site surgery, including the amputation of the wrong body part. Anesthesiologists often use checklists to prepare to give anesthesia, helping make sure the proper equipment and drugs are available, any known allergies or previous untoward reactions are identified, and the correct patient receives the correct care. Blood products are triple-checked to ensure they are appropriate

and compatible for the patient. Surgeons use timeouts just before making the initial incision to double-check the patient's identity, operative site, consent, allergies, preoperative medications given, all needed supplies available (implants, bone plates, drill bits, and so on), and all needed equipment available, among other necessities. Hospital safety protocols also relate to issues such as patient falls, giving patients the wrong dose or wrong medication, and failure to hand wash between patients during rounds. Hospitals also usually have protocols in place to address nonclinical problems, such as fires, bomb threats, intruders, and power outages. It is now common for safety issues to be part of medical staff meeting agendas and various standing committees of the hospital. Through these efforts, the frequency of patient injuries has dropped dramatically.

CULTURE OF SAFETY IN ORAL-MAXILLOFACIAL SURGERY

OMS practices with a culture of safety see several benefits. The incidence of patient injuries decreases, an obvious positive outcome. Injuries not only affect the health and satisfaction of the patient suffering the harm, but can affect a practice's local reputation and be a trigger of legal action. Thus, patient safety is a winning strategy. Workplace injuries are also deleterious to a practice. Doctors and staff injuries on the job often result in lost workdays, a decrease in practice income, and lowered morale. Therefore, a practice that has developed a culture of safety should take steps to make patients and new employees of the practice aware of the high priority the organization places on keeping everyone as safe as possible.[8,9]

The culture of safety in an OMS dentoalveolar practice has several dimensions. These dimensions are as follows:

1. Clinical care safety
2. Intraoffice guest and health care team safety
3. Safety from extraoffice dangers.

Each plays an important role when embracing the culture of safety concept.

CLINICAL CARE SAFETY

OMS offices have a strong track record of taking steps to avoid patient harm in the provision of clinical care. These steps relate to various aspects of patient management. Dentoalveolar surgery–related precautions include ensuring the correct tooth to be removed or surgical site to be operated on is double-checked by the surgeon and assisting staff. This step is similar to the timeout strategy

---

Box 1
Culture of safety definition

A culture of safety is the establishment of organizational behavior in which members of the organization place a high priority on identifying and rectifying safety issues.

used in hospital operating rooms. This step helps slow down what is often a hectic schedule at the moment when haste may lead to critical errors. Other evidence-based safety measures include keeping incisions distal to lower third molars over the lateral cortex of the ascending ramus, avoiding overelevation (retraction) on the lingual aspect of lower third molars, carefully elevating maxillary molar teeth before or instead of using extraction forceps, and carefully measuring the distance over the inferior alveolar canal before the implant site preparation. Rotary equipment is a common threat to patient safety. Such equipment can develop heat in the cutting area and along the shaft capable of burning patient tissue. Irrigation prevents heat accumulation at the surgical site, but not elsewhere on the drill. Recently autoclaved instruments not allowed to properly cool are another source of patient burn injuries. A spinning burr can easily cut tissue outside of the surgical site if allowed to rotate while inserting or removing the drill from the site. Similar unwanted cuts can occur if the surgeon is not focused on the scalpel blade while it moves to and from the planned incision site. Oral and maxillofacial surgeons are trained in numerous other means of lowering the incidence of unplanned surgical injuries.

Anesthetic injuries are also possible. Their prevention usually revolves around careful preparation to manage emergencies and precisely monitoring the patient while anesthetized. Pulse oximeters and end-tidal carbon dioxide monitors are important means of detecting patient hypoxia or bradypnea. When these monitors are added to the surgeon's and assistant's visual monitoring of the anesthetized patient, problems potentially leading to patient injuries are highly unlikely. Preparing for managing anesthetic emergencies is also part of a culture of safety. Again, oral and maxillofacial surgeons typically ensure the ready availability of airway adjuncts, drug reversal agents, and resuscitation equipment and supplies. Checklists can be useful for this task. Regular surgical team emergency drills are another component of emergency preparation. After surgery, clear protocols should be in place for when patients may be moved, how they are monitored during recovery and by whom, and formal criteria for discharge to the care of their escort. Finally, for child patients, long-acting local anesthetics should be avoided.

Medication errors are more likely in a hospital setting simply because of the larger variety and frequency of administration compared with an OMS office. However, oral and maxillofacial surgeons and their team should take similar steps to protect patients. These steps include checking the expiration date of drugs, double-checking that the correct drug and dosage are being administered to the right patient, double-checking that indwelling lines are indeed in a vein before using them for drug administration, and double-checking that patient allergies and other history of adverse drug reactions are documented and reviewed before giving a patient any drug, including prescriptions. Small patients and those under the age of 12 require adjustment of dosages of anesthetic drugs and other medications to avoid untoward reactions.

Patients can also suffer nonphysical injuries when receiving health care. Following HIPPA (Health Insurance Portability and Accountability) regulations will minimize these risks. In addition, because patients often use credit cards to pay for services, office computer equipment should have software in place that lessens the chances of identity theft.

The final aspect of clinical care safety involves being cognizant of and making appropriate care modifications for patients with medical conditions. A well-planned and executed protocol for documenting and updating patient health issues is important to prevent or be prepared to manage medical emergencies affecting ambulatory office patients. This area is another area where having an emergency management case or cart and conducting periodic drills are essential.

INTRAOFFICE GUEST AND HEALTH CARE TEAM SAFETY

Injuries in the OMS office can occur to nonpatients as well. These injuries can affect individuals accompanying patients, delivery people, cleaning crews, and others that fall into the category of office guests. Safety concerns affecting guests typically relate to problems such as wet floors, loose rugs, and other tripping hazards and things located where they might cause head injuries, such as low hanging objects or heavy objects susceptible to falling from elevated sites. Because many patients may have young children accompanying them, office reception areas should be screened to remove items that may risk harm to young guests. Regularly monitoring for all potential hazards is part of an office culture of safety.

Clinical care team safety is another facet of preventing injuries. The OSHA (Occupational Safety and Health Administration) has many regulations in place that mandate certain employee safety practices. The owners of OMS practices are usually well aware of those requirements that include the safe use of chemicals, radiation, and power equipment. In addition, the increase in the use of universal precautions during the 1980s made the wearing of protective garments, masks, and eyewear become routine. Similarly, the adoption of protocols involving the proper use and disposal of sharps has also improved workplace safety. Because back injuries are common in the workplace, protocols for lifting heavy objects or patients should be established. The main thrust of an office seeking to grow a culture of safety for the patient care team is not just to develop safety practices but also to ingrain in team members an unwavering adherence to established protocols and comfort in reminding those forgetting to follow them (**Box 2**).

SAFETY FROM EXTRAOFFICE THREATS

Although complex and time-consuming to establish, creating a culture of safety in the OMS office

---

Box 2
Safety threats in oral-maxillofacial surgery practice

Clinical care examples

   Treatment at wrong site/on wrong tooth

   Nerve damage from incisions, retraction, or power equipment

   Tuberosity fracture

   Soft tissue burns

   Damage outside of surgical field

   Damage to vital structures during implant placement

   Hypoxia during advanced forms of anesthesia

   Drug overdose or incorrect drug used

   Premature discharge after anesthesia

Care team and guest examples

   Tripping and slipping

   Electrical shocks

   Chemical burns

   Radiation overexposure

   Injury from sharps and power equipment

   Contraction of infectious diseases

   Back injuries

External threats

   Tripping and slipping

   Assaults and robberies

   Severe weather

   Floods, earthquakes, and fires

   Electrical outages

---

is usually fully under the control of the surgeon and their staff. Much of this control is lost once patients, guests, and care team members leave the office. An office site controlling its own external walkways and parking facilities does have some control over things such as tripping or slipping hazards and should regularly monitor those parts of the property, including ensuring proper ice and snow removal when applicable. The owners of the practice who identify dangers in public areas near their property, such as broken sidewalks or nonfunctioning street illumination, can alert public agencies to the areas in need of repair. The dangers of external office assaults or robberies on the premises might be mitigated by security fencing, escorts to vehicles, and video monitoring equipment. Other dangers may be totally out of anyone's control, including electrical outages, severe weather, fires, floods, and earthquakes. In these cases, an office with a culture of safety should develop contingency plans of how office staff should react to protect patients and guests, as well as themselves, in the event of an actual or threatening emergency. These protocols should be in writing and known to members of the staff to help minimize the chances of preventable injuries.

ESTABLISHING A CULTURE OF SAFETY

Although protecting patients, guests, and employees from injuries makes perfect sense, establishing a true culture of safety can be challenging. It is easy to take shortcuts in patient care that bypass safety protocols, because many shortcuts take less time and less thought and focus than ensuring safety practices are followed. Employees may not understand or care why a culture of safety is important. Having a culture of safety in place does put the onus on everyone to be vigilant when at the office to look for hazards and take the steps necessary to remove or reduce the risk.

Therefore, it is mandatory that an office's surgeons take the lead in instituting a culture of safety and in continuing to nurture it over the long run. Discussions of safety matters should be a standard agenda item for office meetings. Staff members identifying ways to improve office safety should receive encouragement, and all staff should understand that helping foster office safety is an essential part of their job. Surgeon leaders need to "walk the walk," closely following safety protocols and making it clear by word and deed that safety is an organizational priority.

The OMS dentoalveolar office, like a hospital, can be the site of injuries to patients, guests, and employees. By establishing and promoting an office culture of safety, preventable injuries can be minimized. Like other measures used to manage risk and potential liability, a culture of safety can provide valuable peace of mind to those responsible for ensuring the success of an OMS office.

REFERENCES

1. Hoffman G. The history of car safety. Aol/Autos. 2007. Available at: http://www.autos.aol.com/article/car-safety-history. Accessed April 20, 2015.

2. Treadwell JR, Lucas S, Tsou AY. Surgical checklists: a systemic review of impacts and implementation. BMJ Qual Saf 2014;23:299–318.

3. Gawande A. Complications: a surgeon's note on an imperfect science. New York: Picador; 2002.

4. Gawande A. The checklist manifesto. New York: Picador; 2009.

5. Brennan TA, Leape LL, Laird NM, et al. Incidence of adverse events and negligence in hospitalized patients – results of the Harvard Medical Practice Study I. N Engl J Med 1991;324:370–6.

6. Schamel J. How the checklist came about. Flight Service Station History. 2012. Available at: http://www.atchistory.org/History/checklst.htm. Accessed April 20, 2015.

7. Does improving safety culture affect patient outcomes? The Health Foundation. 2011. Available at: http://www.health.org.uk/public/cms/75/76/313/3078/Does%20improving%20safety%20culture%20affect%20outcomes.pdf?realName=fsu8Va.pdf. Accessed April 20, 2015.

8. Develop a culture of safety. Institute for Healthcare Improvement. Available at: http://www.ihi.org/resources/Pages/Changes/DevelopaCultureofSafety.aspx. Accessed April 20, 2015.

9. Yamalik N, Perea Pérez B. Patient safety and dentistry: what do we need to know? Fundamental patient safety, the safety culture and implementation of patient safety measures in dental practice. Int Dent J 2012;62(2):189–96.

Trigeminal Nerve Injuries
Avoidance and Management of Iatrogenic Injury

Sami A. Nizam II, DMD, MD, Vincent B. Ziccardi, DDS, MD*

KEYWORDS

- Trigeminal nerve injuries • Iatrogenic injury • Dentoalveolar surgery

KEY POINTS

- Neurosensory disturbances after dentoalveolar surgery remain a significant concern for patients and surgeons.
- Mechanisms of trigeminal nerve injures resulting from dentoalveolar injury include surgical endodontic therapy, removal of impacted teeth, local anesthetic nerve blocks, implant placement, bone grafting, and management of oral and maxillofacial pathology.
- Current literature indicates third molar removal has the highest overall risk for injury to either the inferior alveolar nerve or lingual nerve, occurring in 0.4% to 22% of cases.
- Iatrogenic injury to the trigeminal nerve can remain a source of concern and litigation even for the most experienced oral and maxillofacial surgeons.

INTRODUCTION

The specialty of oral and maxillofacial surgery has continued to broaden its scope; however, the most significant aspect of many practices remains dentoalveolar surgery. The specialty's commitment to maintaining excellence and providing the highest standard of care is paramount for patients, and is the overall theme of this issue. Neurosensory disturbances after dentoalveolar surgery remain a significant concern for patients and surgeons. This article focuses on identifying mechanisms of trigeminal nerve injury and their prevalence, pertinent preoperative evaluation, strategies to minimize risk, identification of injury including sensory testing, indications for referral to microsurgeons, and a discussion of medical management options.

Mechanisms of trigeminal nerve injuries resulting from dentoalveolar injury include surgical endodontic therapy, removal of impacted teeth, local anesthetic nerve blocks, implant placement, bone grafting, and management of oral and maxillofacial pathology. Libersa and colleagues[1] conducted a review of insurance claims from 1988 to 1997 in France. They grouped nerve injury patients into one of four groups: (1) surgical procedure (removal of teeth excluding third molars, cysts, and nerve blocks), (2) third molar removal, (3) endodontic treatment, and (4) implant placement. It was determined that third molar removal had the highest incidence of injury (40.8%), followed by endodontic therapy (35.3%), other surgical procedures (20.7%), and implant placement (3.2%). This is consistent with typical clinical practice in which third molar removal is the most commonly performed surgical procedure in most oral and maxillofacial surgery offices. In 2011, Renton and Yilmaz[2] published their study describing causes of 93 lingual nerve injuries and 90 inferior alveolar nerve injuries and reported similar findings to the previously mentioned study. In regards to inferior

Department of Oral and Maxillofacial Surgery, Rutgers University School of Dental Medicine, 110 Bergen Street, Room B854, Newark, NJ 07103-2400, USA
* Corresponding author.
E-mail address: ziccarvb@sdm.rutgers.edu

Oral Maxillofacial Surg Clin N Am 27 (2015) 411–424
http://dx.doi.org/10.1016/j.coms.2015.04.006
1042-3699/15/$ – see front matter © 2015 Elsevier Inc. All rights reserved.

alveolar nerve (IAN) injury, third molar surgery was again the most common (60%), followed by local anesthetic injections (19%), implants (18%), and endodontic surgery (18%). The higher prevalence for implant-related injury likely highlights the increasing prevalence of implant placement by nonsurgeons. They also reviewed lingual nerve injury in their population and found 73% to be caused by third molar removal and 17% by local anesthesia injections.

PREOPERATIVE EVALUATION

As with any surgical procedure, patient evaluation begins with review of chief complaint, medical history, and physical examination. This should be augmented with appropriate imaging studies. After data have been collected, a true appreciation of risks and benefits can be presented to the patient as part of the informed consent process. Patient selection, indicated procedures, risks, and benefits can be discussed with the patient using American Association of Oral and Maxillofacial Surgeons Parameters of Care as a guide.[3]

Current literature indicates third molar removal has the highest overall risk for injury to either the inferior alveolar nerve or lingual nerve, occurring in 0.4% to 22% of cases. This is well appreciated by the oral and maxillofacial surgery community because there is a significant body of research devoted to the issue of trigeminal nerve injury including prevention, assessment, and management. Patients older than age 35 have an increased risk of IAN injury presumably from denser cortical bone, fully developed root structure, concomitant medical conditions, and decreased healing potential. The type of impaction and operator experience correlate with increased risk of nerve injury, specifically depth and angulation of the impactions. The more tissue manipulation and/or bone removal required correlates with increased risk of injury. For instance, there is an increased chance of injury in horizontally impacted teeth when compared with mesioangular, vertical, or distoangular impactions. Third molars removed in the operating room under general anesthesia have also been shown to have increased chance of injury, presumably from increased forces and overall more difficult case selection.[4] The authors have also hypothesized that local anesthetic nerve blocks given to patients under general anesthesia could potentially have an increased incidence of nerve injuries because patients are unable to respond to injections while under general anesthesia. For this reason, the authors do not administer nerve blocks to patients under general anesthesia, but rather use local infiltration techniques.

Panoramic radiograph should be considered a standard of care in the preoperative evaluation of patients with impacted third molars. In 1990, Rood and Shehab[5] published their landmark article correlating panoramic radiographic imaging with potential IAN injury. They described three factors that were considered to indicate high potential for IAN injury because of proximity of the impacted third molar roots with the IAN. These radiographic findings included radiolucency of the IAN canal shadow across the root of the impacted molar, deviation or deflection of the IAN canal, and interruption of the white line delineating the superior and inferior margins of the IAN canal. Two of these signs are present in the panoramic film depicted in **Fig. 1**. Signs that were considered clinically important were deflection of third molar root by canal and narrowing of third molar root. Many studies have confirmed these as reliable indicators of involvement of the IAN and most practitioners still use these criteria in the preoperative evaluation of patients before third molar surgery.[5]

With the advent and availability of cone-beam computed tomography (CBCT), many oral and maxillofacial surgery practices use this advanced imaging modality in the preoperative risk assessment of patients with complex impacted third molars. This is not advocated for the routine evaluation of every third molar patient because of cost and radiation exposure; however, it remains a useful supplementary imaging modality in those patients identified on panoramic radiographs as being high risk for IAN injury because of local pathology or the relative position of the impacted tooth with the IAN canal. Most of the reported

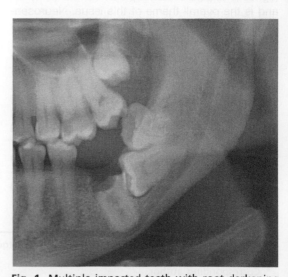

Fig. 1. Multiple impacted teeth with root darkening at the apex of #18 and diversion at the apex of tooth #19 evident on panoramic radiograph.

research focuses on those patients determined to be high risk by Rood's criteria. It is known that exposure or contact of a tooth root with the IAN increases the chance of nerve injury 20% to 30%.[6] Researchers have focused on assessment of decortication of the IAN canal by the root of the third molar as a risk factor. Nakamori and colleagues[7] found that when Rood's criteria were present, there was a greater than 50% chance of decortication of the IAN canal. The group cautioned, however, that teeth that were deemed superimposed and did not meet Rood's criteria still had a 32% chance of demonstrating decortication of the canal. Guerrero and colleagues[8] examined just this group and determined that CBCT is more accurate than panoramic radiographs; however, clinically this did not result in a difference in neurosensory outcome for patients. Selvi and colleagues[9] recently examined the high-risk group of patients and found that in particular, darkening of the root did correlate with cortical perforation on CBCT. Furthermore, a decortication of the canal greater than 3 mm correlated with an increased risk of injury at time of surgery.[9,10] **Fig. 2** presents a sagittal and coronal CT image of the same patient presented in **Fig. 1** that was selected for further imaging based on Rood's criteria.

Proponents of advanced imaging, such as CBCT or traditional CT scanning, state that advanced imaging allows for formulation of surgical plans and therefore avoidance of iatrogenic injury to the nerve. This is highlighted by Umar and colleagues,[11] where 200 teeth demonstrating contact with the IAN on imaging were removed with a 12% incidence of temporary hypoesthesia and no permanent deficits. Opponents argue that there have been no randomized clinical trials demonstrating actual outcome benefit with advanced imaging. In light of current controversy over the role of advanced imaging, the most recent

American Association of Oral and Maxillofacial Surgeons Parameters of Care states "Indications for cone beam computed tomography for routine third molar surgery should be documented before ordering scans and follow the principles of ALARA (as low as reasonably achievable)," essentially leaving the decision to the surgeon's discretion.[3]

Lingual nerve injury during third molar removal occurs at a similar rate of 0.4% to 22% of cases. MRI studies have elucidated the preoperative position of the nerve to be at or above the height of the lingual alveolar crest in 10% of patients and in contact with the lingual plate in 25% of cases in the third molar region.[12,13] **Fig. 3** demonstrates an example where a high lingual nerve was damaged during extraction of tooth #32 and subsequently reconstructed. Anatomic factors, such as lingual angulation of the impacted tooth and need for vertical sectioning, increase the risk of lingual nerve injury.[4] Ultrasound has also recently been described as an alternative imaging modality for assessing the path of the lingual nerve in this region. Benninger and coworkers[14] using cadavers described the path of the nerve as traveling on average 13.2-mm anteriorly from the distolingual aspect of the third molar before it turned inferior and medial to innervate the tongue on ultrasound studies. They additionally reported the nerve being 7.3-mm inferior to the lingual alveolar crest on average, with this number remaining similar between dentate and edentulous patients. This 13.2-mm anterior travel along the lingual cortex places it in intimate contact with the second molar site and provides a route for potential iatrogenic injury during third molar surgery.[14]

Preoperative evaluation for implant patients also begins with thorough physical examination. Bone stock availability and bone defects can be appreciated through bimanual palpation. If a thin ridge is encountered and bone height will be removed for implant placement, this vertical change needs

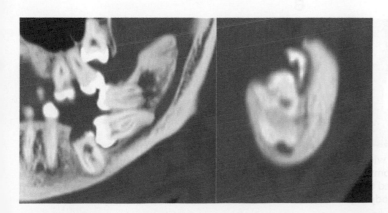

Fig. 2. CT scan images of the patient in **Fig. 1**. Note the loss of decortication of the canal on teeth #18 and #19. The inferior alveolar nerve is noted to be present in the notched apex of impacted tooth.

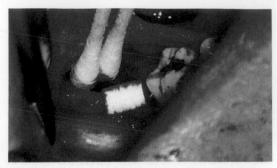

Fig. 3. Example of lingual nerve above the lingual crest (10% incidence), which was subsequently injured during extraction of tooth #32. The nerve has been repaired after excision of neuroma and covered with Neuragen collagen conduit from Integra Life Sciences (Plainsboro, NJ).

to be factored into the final height of bone available for implant placement. As with third molar removal, panoramic imaging remains clinically useful for the initial evaluation of implant patients with the understanding that distortion can create inaccuracy of up to 25%. Standardization can be accomplished by placing a known-size metallic object in the area of interest and accounting for distortion based on actual measurements of the metallic object. Once the radiograph is taken, a simple conversion formula can be used to determine actual bone height ([radiographic bone height/radiographic marker size] x [N/actual marker size], where N is actual bone height). A 2-mm margin of safety should be minimally maintained above the IAN canal. If this margin is not available or poor visualization of the nerve is present, then an advanced imaging technique, such as CBCT, should be considered.[15] **Fig. 4** shows an instance where a 2-mm safety margin was not maintained at time of implant placement. Alternatively, bone augmentation of the deficient ridge is an option to be discussed with patients in re-

establishing bone heights for better mechanical stability of implants. CBCT and other implant planning software could also be used to position implants buccal or lingual relative to the IAN canal if indicated.

A similar algorithm can be developed for implants placed in the mental foramen region, the only difference being the placement of implants anterior to the foramen because of a possible anterior loop of the nerve before exit from the bony canal. Greenstein and colleagues[16] reviewed the literature on this subject and found a wide variance of not only presence of the anterior loop but also its distance when it exists. If a planned implant osteotomy encroaches within 2-mm superiorly or anterior to the mental foramen, they suggest two options: CBCT or surgically probing the canal with a Nabers 2N probe at time of surgery. The key to probing is to probe the distal aspect of the foramen. If it is not patent, this means the nerve enters from an anterior to posterior region signifying an anterior loop. This same procedure cannot be performed probing anterior in the foramen because the incisive portion of the canal will be probed. The authors advocate maintaining a distance of 5-mm anterior to the visible mental foramina to avoid injuries to the anterior loop of the IAN.

Planning for periradicular endodontic surgery in the posterior mandible starts as described previously with physical examination including neurologic examination. Although rare, numerous reports exist of periapical infection and inflammation producing temporary neurosensory disturbances. This may occur because of roots of the premolars and distal root of the second molar having close proximity to the IAN with inflammation or pathology at the apex.[17] This provides clinical information as to the indication of close involvement of the IAN and the possibility of a more serious cause, such as malignancy, to be ruled out with

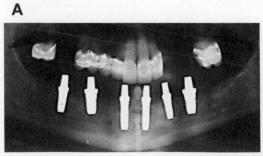
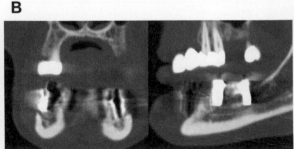

Fig. 4. (*A*) Panoramic image of patient with bilateral IAN damage caused by improper planning before placement of ceramic implants. Also note osteotomy shadows bilaterally, which represent temporary implants removed by secondary surgeon that also contributed to nerve injury. (*B*) Same patient demonstrating bilateral compression of the IAN at the mental foramen and body region.

laboratory assessment of pathologic tissues. Velvart and coworkers[18] examined a series of 78 patients scheduled for periradicular endodontic surgery and found definitive identification of the IAN in only half of these patients and evidence of the periapical lesion in only 61 of the 78 patients. They suggested if the mandibular canal cannot be detected in imaging or is in close proximity, CT scan should be used to delineate the existing anatomy and provide the added benefit of elucidating the three-dimensional anatomy around the tooth apex.[18] **Fig. 5** depicts the postoperative panoramic radiograph of a patient who underwent apicoectomy of tooth #19 with injury to the IAN.

SURGICAL STRATEGIES FOR AVOIDANCE OF INJURIES

After risk stratification using the previously mentioned methods, discussion with the patient occurs to decide on the particular surgical procedure to be performed. If the patient fits into a high-risk category for any of the previously mentioned reasons and there is no active pathology associated with impacted teeth, partial intentional odontectomy or orthodontic extrusion should be considered. Surgeon experience has also been found linked to lower incidence of postoperative neurosensory deficits.[4] For the experienced surgeon, a traditional extraction may still be attempted with good outcome if the prior stated algorithm is used and no absolute contraindications to extraction exist.[11] The authors often use this approach after advanced imaging with surgery performed in the operating room under general anesthesia to allow potential repair of any witnessed nerve injury at the time of surgery. These cases often demonstrate exposure of the nerve

intraoperatively, which can be protected by covering with resorbable gelatin sponge.

For routine extractions, a plan is formulated that allows the least amount of force, trauma, and development of postoperative edema to be placed on the neurovascular bundle. Preoperative steroids have been found in small studies to attenuate sensory disturbances after extraction of third molars.[19] Additionally, nonsteroidal anti-inflammatory drugs (NSAIDs), in particular diclofenac, have been shown by Shanti and coworkers[20] 2013 to attenuate post–sciatic nerve injury in a rat model. The combination of dexamethasone and diclofenac was studied in 2005 with a preoperative dose of 8-mg dexamethasone and 50-mg diclofenac and a postoperative dose of 4-mg dexamethasone and continued 5-mg diclofenac two times a day for 5 days. The combination was found to be synergistic when compared with either agent alone and provided statistically significant decrease in short-term pain and swelling.[21] Prophylactic antibiotics have recently been demonstrated in the Cochrane database to prevent complications after extractions of third molars.[22] In light of the data, and the added benefits of patient comfort, it seems reasonable that a preoperative dose of steroids, NSAID, and antibiotic may be advised before undertaking complex third molar impaction surgery.

Complex impacted tooth removal may require the use of releasing incisions. On designing the incisions, the surgeon must also pay particular attention to the lingual crest because of variability in the position of the lingual nerve necessitating a distobuccal release to avoid nerve injury.[13] In rare circumstances, the nerve may take a path across the retromolar pad, in which case lingual nerve injury is almost unavoidable in even the most skilled hands. Once a surgical flap is developed, a subperiosteal dissection is undertaken. If the preoperative plan dictates need for distal bone removal, a lingual flap may be retracted for better visualization and protection of the lingual nerve. This technique has been shown to result in higher temporary neurosensory disturbance but no increase in long-term disturbance (something that should be disclosed during the consent process).[23] The surgical plan is then carried out with appropriate troughing of the bone to the level of the cementoenamel junction to allow for visualization and performance of sectioning with caution not to encroach on the lingual plate. Once the crown is sectioned and removed, roots can be delivered with minimal force to allow for copious socket irrigation. A visual assessment of the socket is then undertaken noting any lingual perforation or exposure of the IAN neurovascular bundle, which should also be noted in

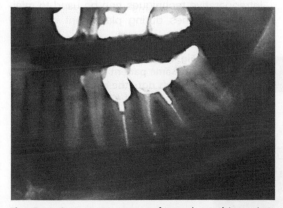

Fig. 5. Apicoectomy was performed on this patient without the use of advanced imaging despite close proximity to the IAN nerve resulting in nerve injury.

the patient record. It may be advised to document pertinent negative findings at this time, such as intact lingual plate, no bone fractures, no active bleeding from socket, and no visualization of the IAN noted. **Fig. 6** presents intraoperative photographs of the same patient in **Figs. 1** and **2**. Wide access was obtained with releasing incisions in an operative room setting with the patient under general anesthesia. Note the exposure of the IAN as preoperative CT predicted. The site was reconstructed using gelatin sponge as a protective barrier over the nerve and then grafted with allogeneic bone and finally collagen membrane.

If control of hemorrhage becomes necessary, the appropriate agent must be selected. Alkan and colleagues[24] reviewed four commonly used hemostatic agents and found oxidized regenerated cellulose to cause an increase in compound action potentials and decrease in nerve conduction velocity at 1 hour, with full sensory recovery by 4 weeks. They found a gelatin sponge to demonstrate an increased compound action potential at 4 weeks, although their sponge was coated with silver potentially causing this effect. They cautioned against the use of bone wax because of case reports of chronic inflammation and embolization to the lungs. They concluded that bovine collagen was the safest agent in regards to adverse effects on neural function. Collagen conduits are a popular choice for nerve entubulization techniques clinically.

Once hemostasis is obtained, a single suture should be placed for partial closure distal to the second molar. A review of recent literature revealed this to be the best overall closure method in regards to edema and ease of application.[25] One must also be aware of proximity to the lingual nerve and not take an excessive bite of lingual tissue to avoid incorporating the lingual nerve with suturing, which can directly damage the nerve with the needle, and potentially compressing the nerve after tie down of the suture.[26]

Partial intentional odontectomy or coronectomy provides another option (discussed elsewhere in this issue). Contraindications for intentional partial odontectomy include significant medical comorbidities, such as immunocompromization, patients planned for or having received radiation therapy, patients with poorly controlled diabetes, and the presence of local pathology that contradicts use of this technique.[27] Horizontally impacted teeth have been reported as a relative contraindication, although a recent article by Monaco and colleagues[28] reporting on this technique found no complications when treating horizontal impactions.

Orthodontic extrusion is another potential option for extraction of third molars at high risk; however, the authors have minimal experience with this techniques and it has had limited review in the literature. Orthodontic anchorage is first obtained with banding of the first molars and a stainless steel lingual arch wire welded too it. The anchorage is further strengthened with a stainless steel sectional wire from second molar to first bicuspid. Tooth angulation dictates bracket position. Vertical or distal angulated teeth require bracket placement on the occlusal surface centered in an axial position. Mesially or horizontally inclined teeth require bracketing on the distal surface of the crown and possibly stripping of a portion of the crown. Regardless of impaction type, advanced imaging is necessary to appreciate vector of forces required to erupt the roots away from the canal. After 1 week of soft tissue healing, a cantilever wire is placed off the buccal tube on the first molar to the bracket placed on the impacted third molar. This is then adjusted every 4 to 6 weeks until the tooth is extruded. A panoramic radiograph is then taken once clinical extrusion has been confirmed. Standard third molar impaction techniques can be used once the risk of injury to the IAN is minimized.[29]

Intraoperative techniques can be used to minimize nerve injuries during placement of dental

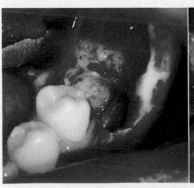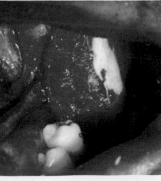

Fig. 6. Intraoperative photographs of the same patient in **Figs. 1** and **2**. On the left note the exposure of the IAN at the apex of #18 as predicted by CT scan. The image to the right shows allograft placed over gelatin sponge, which was used as a protective barrier of the IAN. The patient underwent a short period of maxillomandibular fixation and experienced no neurosensory deficits postoperatively.

implants in the mandible. This starts with local anesthesia techniques where some have advocated the use of infiltration versus a block, allowing the patient to respond to pain if there is encroachment on the nerve.[30] If a flap is being reflected and it is in the second molar region, the practitioner must be cognizant of the potential for proximity to the lingual nerve.[14] Careful retraction of the flap in the mental nerve region and skeletonization of the nerve as it exits the mandible may also be necessary to avoid traction injuries. During osteotomy preparation, use of periapical radiographs with marking pins has been shown to decrease the chance of neurovascular encroachment, particular in cases of marginal vertical height.[31] Some also advocate the use of stoppers on osteotomy burs to avoid overpenetration.[15] Osteotomy sites should be palpated with blunt probe to ensure there is no decortication of the nerve canal. Surgical guides have been demonstrated to increase accuracy, although these guides must be properly positioned to avoid inaccuracy when transferring from the virtual plan to the patient. A 2-mm safety zone should still be followed to allow for any potential inaccuracies. Thermal injury can occur even without direct penetration because of lack of appropriate irrigation or high-drill speeds. If graft materials are placed and there is decortication of the canal, this material may be mechanically pressed into the canal causing nerve injuries. Finally, at the time of implant insertion, the implant must not be placed beyond the apical extent of the osteotomy by countersinking if the IAN is known to be close apically.[32]

Apical surgery begins with review of existing imaging. Landmarks should be identified to help guide the surgeon intraoperatively and maintain safe distances from the IAN and mental foramen. Three incision designs can be used: (1) sulcular, (2) papilla sparing, and (3) a semilunar flap.[33] Typically releasing incisions are used with the first two and these should be planned at least one tooth anterior or posterior to the identified mental foramen. The dissection for all incisions should then be subperiosteal and if near the mental nerve this structure should be identified and protected to avoid iatrogenic injury during instrumentation. Access to the periapical lesion and root should be obtained using anatomic references that were selected before surgery. Caution must be exercised when instrumenting the cavity being cognizant of anatomic danger zones mentioned previously. Once the periapical lesion has been removed, hemostasis is achieved using known hemostatic agents.[24] If the nerve is exposed, a resorbable collagen barrier should be placed over the nerve to provide a barrier from the root end filling material. In an in vitro model, mineral trioxide aggregate was found to be the only root end filling material that was incapable of inducing neurotoxicity even while setting.[34] Because of its favorable biocompatibility it provides an excellent material choice when the IAN is in close proximity. If guided bone regeneration is planned and graft material is placed at the apex one must ensure it is not compacted into the canal. **Fig. 7** depicts intraoperative photographs of the same patient in **Fig. 5**. The nerve had presumably been damaged from aggressive curettage or rotary instrumentation at the time of injury. Foreign body was noted within the resultant scar tissue and submitted to pathology.

Although no preoperative evaluation can avoid local anesthetic-related nerve injury, injection technique can play a role. When performing mental nerve or inferior alveolar nerve blocks, the surgeon should aspirate before injection. If a patient reports an immediate jolt or shock-like sensation, the needle should also be withdrawn and redirected to avoid intraneural injection. The event should be documented in the chart to help differentiate cause in the event a nerve injury occurs.[32] The use of high-concentration local anesthetics should be avoided, and multiple blocks if at all possible. In particular 4% prilocaine and 4% articaine are 7.3% and 3.6% more likely to cause paresthesia when used for IAN nerve blocks.[35] Additionally, these agents have a higher chance of producing neuropathic pain compared with other commonly used local anesthetic agents.[36]

WHEN INJURY OCCURS

Unfortunately, despite the best preparation and surgical techniques, injuries may still occur. Time

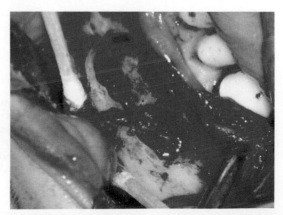

Fig. 7. Damaged IAN nerve at apicoectomy site #19 shown in **Fig. 5**. The nerve appears to be damaged from either rotary instrumentation or aggressive curettage. A foreign body was also noted within the scar tissue and sent for pathologic examination.

from injury dictates actions that can be taken. Witnessed or open injuries mandate immediate or delayed early intervention depending on surgeon skill level. If the patient is in the operating room and appropriate equipment is available, immediate repair may be attempted. If not, the ends of the nerve can be tagged with nonresorbable suture, such as nylon or polypropylene, and the wound closed. Note is made of the site and type of injury and prompt referral can be made to a microneurosurgeon.[26] Prior research has shown benefit to anti-inflammatory medications following acute nerve injury, and consideration should be given to a steroid, NSAIDs, or both.[20]

Most nerve injuries, however, are not witnessed and are noted at postoperative follow-up. The key to ensuring the best overall patient outcome is identification of mechanism, appropriate neurosensory testing, and timely surgical intervention if necessary. An algorithm is provided in **Fig. 8** that may provide guidance to the practitioner faced

with a patient who returns with a postoperative neurosensory deficit.

First and foremost, a baseline complete neurosensory examination is conducted and documented in the chart. This begins with history and a description of the sensory deficit or pain. It must first be classified as painful or unpleasant (dysesthesia) or absent, decreased, or altered (paresthesia, hypoesthesia, or anesthesia). Constant pain is usually a result of a long-term injury that has resulted from lack of afferent input from the periphery (differentiation) and is seen in patients with neuroma formation. If pain is intermittent, one must determine if pain is stimulated or merely spontaneous and the length of each episode. A visual analog scale is then used to quantify the pain on a scale of 1 to 10. The patient should be questioned what if any pain medications have been attempted and if so what their effects have been. If the patient's complaint is caused by decreased sensation it should be quantified

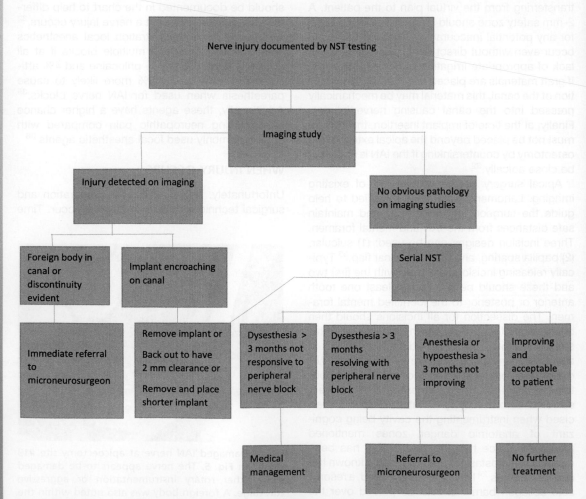

Fig. 8. Trigeminal nerve injury algorithm. NST, neurosensory testing.

on a level of 1 to 10 and compared with the opposite side. For either type of injury, interference with activates of daily living should be documented. Of special note, if a lingual nerve injury has occurred, alteration of taste sensation (paraguesia) should be noted.[26]

After the chief complaint and symptoms have been elucidated, attention is next directed at physical examination. The patient should be seated comfortably and all tests are administered with the patient's eyes closed in a quiet environment. The contralateral normal side is always tested first to establish baselines. The examination starts with mapping of the altered region. This can be done by using the wisp of a cotton-tip applicator in a brush stroke fashion and having the patient raise his or her hand when they no longer sense the cotton. This is then marked and the process is repeated from different directions until the area is marked in its entirety. Photographic documentation can also be taken at this time. At this point, neurosensory testing differs if the patient suffers from anesthesia/paresthesia versus dysesthesia.[4]

If the patient has reduced or no sensation, levels of function are tested in a stepwise approach. Level A testing evaluates larger-diameter A alpha and A beta fibers that are 5 to 12 μm in diameter. This is performed implementing a cotton swab with the cotton drawn into a wisp. Testing is carried out by applying 10 strokes on the normal side and the patient is asked to determine the direction of stroke for each. This process is then repeated on the altered side and results are once again recorded by documenting how many out of the 10 attempts were correctly identified. A score of 9/10 or greater is considered normal. Two-point discrimination is then performed using a Boley gauge or college pliers and a millimeter ruler. The normal side is again tested first by starting with the calipers at zero and lightly touching the area. The patient is asked to identify if this feels as one or two objects. The distance is then incrementally widened until the patient can discriminate two separate points. After this the process is repeated on the side of pathology in similar fashion. Within the inferior alveolar nerve and lingual nerve distributions the patient should have two-point discrimination of 4 mm and 3 mm, respectively. Because there is a large variation from patient to patient, numbers should be correlated to the contralateral nonpathologic side. If the patient has normal responses, the examination need not continue. If abnormal responses are recorded the examiner moves to level B testing.[37]

Level B testing measures the smaller A beta fibers of approximately 4- to 8-μm diameter, which provide static light touch sensation. These fibers are evaluated by lightly touching the skin without indentation with the wooden end of a cotton swab. If the patient cannot feel the contact, the pressure is then increased and the skin is lightly indented. If this can be felt at the higher threshold it is recorded as felt, however, at a higher threshold. If sensation is still not present even at the higher threshold then this is recorded and the examiner moves on to level C testing. Alternatively and more accurately, Semmes-Weinstein filaments may be used. These are a graded set of filaments with increasing pressures required to deform each filament. The filaments can be used in stepwise fashion to accurately assess the patient's threshold for detection.[37,38]

Level C testing measures response to noxious stimulus, which are carried by scantily myelinated A delta fibers or nonmyelinated C fibers. Testing is similar to level B in that initially light contact is made with a dental needle. If the patient does not feel this, contact is then made once again, however this time slightly indenting the skin. If the patient feels this it is recorded as an abnormal response. If the patient does not feel this it is also recorded; however, further pressure need not be applied. Further testing by thermal means is not necessary; however, it may provide insight into the exact damaged fibers. Ethyl chloride spray provides cold stimulus and heat can be applied with warmed gutta-percha or warm water dipped cotton-tip applicators. The results of these tests are then recorded and the patient is diagnosed as being normal, mildly impaired, moderately impaired, severely impaired, or anesthetic. Degrees of impairment can be ascertained from performance at each level of testing using Zuniga and Essik's algorithm seen in **Fig. 9**.[4,37,39]

If the patient suffers from dysesthesia, the three levels are again examined; however, in this context, all three levels are always examined regardless of outcome at any specific level. The goal of this examination is to identify the type of dysesthesia. Starting with level A, testing is carried out as before by stroking the region with a cotton wisp. If the patient experiences pain that stops on removal of the wisp, this is termed allodynia or abnormal pain response to unpainful stimulus that ceases with removal of stimulus. Level B is used to reveal if the patient has hyperpathia, which is present if the patient has delayed-onset pain, increased intensity on repeated stimuli, or pain that continues after the stimulus ends. Level C testing tests for hyperalgesia. As before, a dental needle is used at a normal threshold to evoke pain and a slightly higher threshold if no reaction takes place. If the patient has pain out of proportion to the examination on

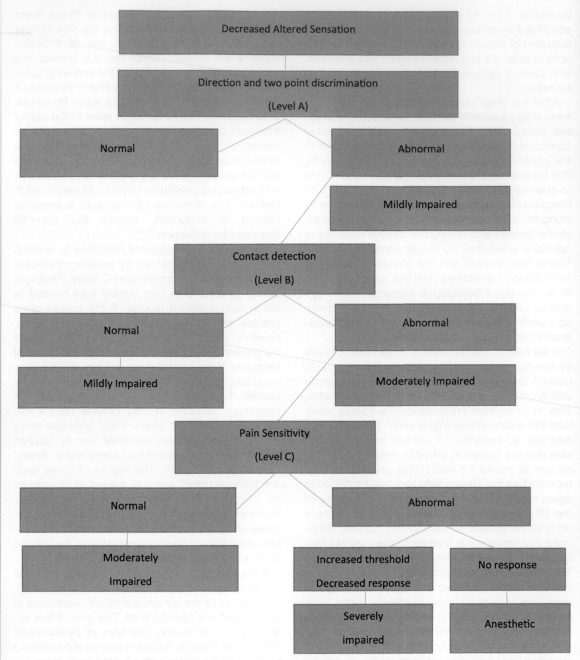

Fig. 9. Grading algorithm for evaluating trigeminal nerve injury by Zuniga and Essik. (*From* Lieblich SE. Endodontic surgery. Dent Clin North Am 2012;56(1):121–32, viii–ix; with permission.)

the contralateral nonpathologic side this is considered hyperalgesia.[37]

Diagnostic nerve blocks may serve as a useful adjunct in localizing the lesion in a patient who is dysesthetic. The blocks can be administered first more peripherally and then more centrally to help locate the lesion. Failure of the local anesthetic block to eradicate symptomatology may indicate that the nerve was not blocked, collateral macro

sprouting has occurred from adjacent nerves, or there is a central mechanism to the pain. If, however, the pain is relieved by diagnostic nerve block, microsurgery may be indicated.[4]

After confirmation of nerve injury, classification, and documentation of injury, one may return to the beginning of the algorithm in **Fig. 8.** The next step is to obtain imaging, which may start with a panoramic radiograph to identify if any obvious pathology is evident. If suspicion exists and a possible mechanical injury is detected, advanced imaging, such as CBCT or traditional CT, may be obtained. If this confirms the suspicion and there is loss of continuity of the canal or encroachment by foreign body, a referral should be made to a microneurosurgeon as soon as possible. If an implant is encroaching on the canal this should be backed out or removed as soon as possible. **Fig. 10** shows the same patient with IAN injury shown in **Fig. 4** at time of surgery. Unfortunately, the implants were not removed at time of identification of injury, relegating her to surgical exploration and repair of the nerve. At this time no reliable method is available for lingual nerve imaging; however, with the advent of 3-T MRI, new imaging sequences, and advanced ultrasound, this may soon be a possibility.

If no obvious pathology is noted, the patient should start a regimen of serial neurosensory testing along with NSAIDS and possible consideration for corticosteroids. An identical examination should be performed at each appointment to allow for comparison over time. Follow-up schedule should include examinations at 1 week, and 1, 2, and 3 months. Controversy still remains as to optimal time for surgical intervention. What is known is that 75% of iatrogenic injuries to the third division of the trigeminal nerve recover without intervention.[40] Perhaps one of the best in vitro studies to date was performed by Jääskeläinen and colleagues[41] in 2004. They intraoperatively monitored 40 IAN nerves during bilateral sagittal split osteotomy (BSSO). They found that simple demyelinating injuries recovered to baseline on neurophysiologic testing within 3 months of injury.

For the reasons described previously, serial neurosensory testing is performed until the 3-month point and a decision is made as to need for surgical intervention. If the patient has no return of sensation, minimal return that is not improving, or dysesthesia that is responsive to peripheral blockade, a referral to a microneurosurgeon is prudent at this time. Our own results have shown statistically significant better sensory outcomes if repair is conducted before 6 months and in particular for IAN injury. Additionally, it has been shown that after 3 months, a complex array of central and peripheral changes that are unlikely to respond to surgical manipulation may occur.[42] This 3-month referral decision point allows for examination, consent, and scheduling within 6 months by a microneurosurgeon. If the patient is experiencing continued improvement, the patient is then followed on a monthly schedule and reassessed when no further improvement occurs or 12 months have been reached. Conflicting data exist in regards to late repair of the IAN and lingual nerve. Good outcomes have been noted in some studies even after the 12-month mark, whereas others note drastic decreases in success.[43,44] Because conflicting evidence is present at this time, it seems prudent to respect wound healing physiology and avoid the irreversible scaring that affects neural tracts by staging any delayed intervention by no later than 1 year. **Fig. 11** depicts a case of late repair. Large neuroma and scar tissue formation is evident requiring resection of a large portion of the lingual nerve and subsequent cadaveric nerve graft (AxoGen, Alachua, FL).

Dysesthesia that is unresponsive to peripheral nerve blocks is likely caused in part by central mechanisms, and surgical repair may not be indicated (see **Fig. 8**). Benoliel and coworkers[45] recently published a review article on this subject detailing terminology, mechanisms, and treatment. They suggested the term painful traumatic trigeminal neuropathy to describe painful lesions

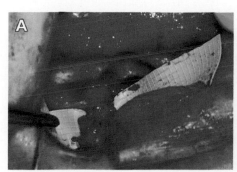 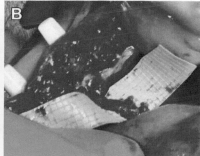

Fig. 10. This is the same patient in **Fig. 3** who suffered bilateral IAN damage during implant placement. Unfortunately the nerves were not decompressed immediately after identification of injury. (*A*) Right IAN after resection of nonviable segment and primary neurorrhaphy and before Axoguard (AxoGen, Alachua, FL) entubulization. (*B*) The left IAN suffered less damage and required only external and internal decompression on exploration.

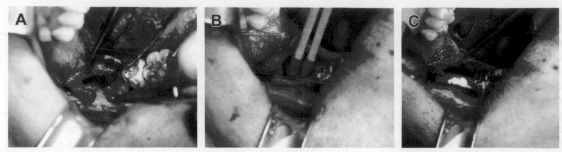

Fig. 11. (*A*) A late lingual nerve repair. Note a large neuroma and large amount of perineural scar tissue formation. (*B*) Because of the condition of the proximal and distal stump a large amount of nerve tissue was excised to allow viable tissue neurorrhaphy. A cadaveric nerve graft (AxoGen) was placed. (*C*) The nerve graft was then surrounded with a Neuragen collagen conduit (Integra Life Sciences) to protect from further perineural scar tissue ingrowth.

postsurgically. Their evidence-based treatment algorithm is seen in **Fig. 12**. After someone has been diagnosed with painful traumatic trigeminal neuropathy, a decision is made to start the patient on tricyclic antidepressants (TCA) or selective norepinephrine receptor inhibitors (duloxetine) versus gabapentin or pregabalin. Amitriptyline remains the drug of choice; however, TCAs have multiple side effects because of their activity at multiple receptors (cholinergic, alpha, histamine,

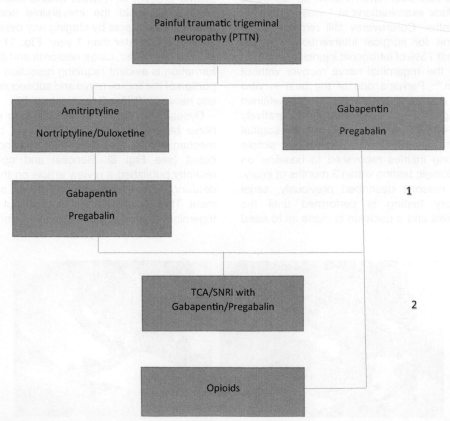

Fig. 12. Stepped approach for treatment of painful traumatic trigeminal neuropathy. (*1*) If anticonvulsants fail strong consideration should be given for combining a selective norepinephrine receptor inhibitor (SNRI). (*2*) If this is contraindicated consideration should be given to opioids. TCA, tricyclic antidepressant. (*From* Zuniga JR, LaBanc JP. Advances in microsurgical nerve repair. J Oral Maxillofac Surg 1993;51(1 Suppl 1):62–8; with permission.)

and so forth) and may be contraindicated or poorly tolerated by patients. Selective norepinephrine receptor inhibitors address one of the TCA mechanisms of action but have been found to be less effective. The newer antiepileptic drugs including gabapentin or pregabalin have a more benign side effect profile and may be started in patients who refuse TCAs or have a contraindication. If either class fails, then the other class is tried. If this fails, then combination therapy is instituted with an agent from each class. If this again fails, opioids may be considered. Unfortunately, even with this stepped approach only 25% of patients experience 30% or greater improvement in symptoms.[46] Of note, these drugs can be used in the management of patients where surgery is indicated to help reduce further central and peripheral sensitization.

SUMMARY

Iatrogenic injury to the trigeminal nerve can remain a source of concern and litigation even for the most experienced oral and maxillofacial surgeons. This article provides the most up-to-date evidence-based recommendations for identification, prevention, and management of these injuries to provide the highest level of patient care. Through this, the specialty can maintain excellence in dentoalveolar surgery.

REFERENCES

1. Libersa P, Savignat M, Tonnel A. Neurosensory disturbances of the inferior alveolar nerve: a retrospective study of complaints in a 10-year period. J Oral Maxillofac Surg 2007;65(8):1486–9.
2. Renton T, Yilmaz Z. Profiling of patients presenting with posttraumatic neuropathy of the trigeminal nerve. J Orofac Pain 2011;25(4):333–44.
3. Carlson ER, Sims PG. Preface to the fifth edition. AAOMS Parameters of Care 2012. J Oral Maxillofac Surg 2012;70(11 Suppl 3):e1–11.
4. Ziccardi VB, Zuniga JR. Nerve injuries after third molar removal. Oral Maxillofac Surg Clin North Am 2007;19(1):105–15, vii.
5. Rood JP, Shehab BA. The radiological prediction of inferior alveolar nerve injury during third molar surgery. Br J Oral Maxillofac Surg 1990;28(1):20–5.
6. Tay AB, Go WS. Effect of exposed inferior alveolar neurovascular bundle during surgical removal of impacted lower third molars. J Oral Maxillofac Surg 2004;62(5):592–600.
7. Nakamori K, Fujiwara K, Miyazaki A, et al. Clinical assessment of the relationship between the third molar and the inferior alveolar canal using

8. panoramic images and computed tomography. J Oral Maxillofac Surg 2008;66(11):2308–13.
8. Guerrero ME, Nackaerts O, Beinsberger J, et al. Inferior alveolar nerve sensory disturbance after impacted third molar evaluation using cone beam computed tomography and panoramic radiography: a pilot study. J Oral Maxillofac Surg 2012;70:2264–70.
9. Selvi F, Dodson TB, Nattestad A, et al. Factors that are associated with injury to the inferior alveolar nerve in high-risk patients after removal of third molars. Br J Oral Maxillofac Surg 2013;51(8):868–73.
10. Susarla SM, Sidhu HK, Avery LL, et al. Does computed tomographic assessment of inferior alveolar canal cortical integrity predict nerve exposure during third molar surgery? J Oral Maxillofac Surg 2010;68(6):1296–303.
11. Umar G, Obisesan O, Bryant C, et al. Elimination of permanent injuries to the inferior alveolar nerve following surgical intervention of the "high risk" third molar. Br J Oral Maxillofac Surg 2013;51(4):353–7.
12. Behnia H, Kheradvar A, Shahrokhi M. An anatomic study of the lingual nerve in the third molar region. J Oral Maxillofac Surg 2000;58(6):649–51 [discussion: 652–3].
13. Miloro M, Halkias LE, Slone HW, et al. Assessment of the lingual nerve in the third molar region using magnetic resonance imaging J Oral Maxillofac Surg 1997;55(2):134–7.
14. Benninger B, Kloenne J, Horn JL. Clinical anatomy of the lingual nerve and identification with ultrasonography. Br J Oral Maxillofac Surg 2013;51(6):541–4.
15. Alhassani AA, AlGhamdi AS. Inferior alveolar nerve injury in implant dentistry: diagnosis, causes, prevention, and management. J Oral Implantol 2010;36(5):401–7.
16. Greenstein G, Tarnow D. The mental foramen and nerve: clinical and anatomical factors related to dental implant placement: a literature review. J Periodontol 2006;77(12):1933–43.
17. von Ohle C, ElAyouti A. Neurosensory impairment of the mental nerve as a sequel of periapical periodontitis: case report and review. Oral Surg Oral Med Oral Pathol Oral Radiol Endod 2010;110(4):e84.
18. Velvart P, Hecker H, Tillinger G. Detection of the apical lesion and the mandibular canal in conventional radiography and computed tomography. Oral Surg Oral Med Oral Pathol Oral Radiol Endod 2001;92(6):682–8.
19. Barron RP, Benoliel R, Zeltser R, et al. Effect of dexamethasone and dipyrone on lingual and inferior alveolar nerve hypersensitivity following third molar extractions: preliminary report. J Orofac Pain 2004;18(1):62–8.
20. Shanti RM, Khan J, Eliav E, et al. Is there a role for a collagen conduit and anti-inflammatory agent in the

management of partial peripheral nerve injuries? J Oral Maxillofac Surg 2013;71(6):1119–25.

21. Bamgbose BO, Akinwande JA, Adeyemo WL, et al. Effects of co-administered dexamethasone and diclofenac potassium on pain, swelling and trismus following third molar surgery. Head Face Med 2005;1:11.

22. Lodi G, Figini L, Sardella A, et al. Antibiotics to prevent complications following tooth extractions. Cochrane Database Syst Rev 2012;(11):CD003811.

23. Pichler JW, Beirne OR. Lingual flap retraction and prevention of lingual nerve damage associated with third molar surgery: a systematic review of the literature. Oral Surg Oral Med Oral Pathol Oral Radiol Endod 2001;91(4):395–401.

24. Alkan A, Inal S, Yildirim M, et al. The effects of hemostatic agents on peripheral nerve function: an experimental study. J Oral Maxillofac Surg 2007;65(4): 630–4.

25. Osunde OD, Adebola RA, Omeje UK. Management of inflammatory complications in third molar surgery: a review of the literature. Afr Health Sci 2011;11(3): 530–7.

26. Meyer RA, Bagheri SC. Nerve injuries from mandibular third molar removal. Atlas Oral Maxillofac Surg Clin North Am 2011;19(1):63–78.

27. Gady J, Fletcher MC. Coronectomy: indications, outcomes, and description of technique. Atlas Oral Maxillofac Surg Clin North Am 2013;21(2):221–6.

28. Monaco G, de Santis G, Gatto MR, et al. Coronectomy: a surgical option for impacted third molars in close proximity to the inferior alveolar nerve. J Am Dent Assoc 2012;143(4):363–9.

29. Alessandri Bonetti G, Bendandi M, Laino L, et al. Orthodontic extraction: riskless extraction of impacted lower third molars close to the mandibular canal. J Oral Maxillofac Surg 2007;65(12): 2580–6.

30. Heller AA, Shankland WE 2nd. Alternative to the inferior alveolar nerve block anesthesia when placing mandibular dental implants posterior to the mental foramen. J Oral Implantol 2001;27(3):127–33.

31. Burstein J, Mastin C, Le B. Avoiding injury to the inferior alveolar nerve by routine use of intraoperative radiographs during implant placement. J Oral Implantol 2008;34(1):34–8.

32. Bagheri SC, Meyer RA. Management of mandibular nerve injuries from dental implants. Atlas Oral Maxillofac Surg Clin North Am 2011;19(1):47–61.

33. Lieblich SE. Endodontic surgery. Dent Clin North Am 2012;56(1):121–32, viii–ix.

34. Asrari M, Lobner D. In vitro neurotoxic evaluation of root-end-filling materials. J Endod 2003;29(11): 743–6.

35. Garisto GA, Gaffen AS, Lawrence HP, et al. Occurrence of paresthesia after dental local anesthetic administration in the United States. J Am Dent Assoc 2010;141(7):836–44.

36. Renton T, Yilmaz Z, Gaballah K. Evaluation of trigeminal nerve injuries in relation to third molar surgery in a prospective patient cohort. Recommendations for prevention. Int J Oral Maxillofac Surg 2012;41(12): 1509–18.

37. Meyer RA, Bagheri SC. Clinical evaluation of peripheral trigeminal nerve injuries. Atlas Oral Maxillofac Surg Clin North Am 2011;19(1):15–33.

38. Poort LJ, van Neck JW, van der Wal KG. Sensory testing of inferior alveolar nerve injuries: a review of methods used in prospective studies. J Oral Maxillofac Surg 2009;67(2):292–300.

39. Zuniga JR, Essick GK. A contemporary approach to the clinical evaluation of trigeminal nerve injuries. Oral Maxillofac Surg Clin North Am 1992;4:353–67.

40. Zuniga JR, LaBanc JP. Advances in microsurgical nerve repair. J Oral Maxillofac Surg 1993;51(1 Suppl 1):62–8.

41. Jääskeläinen SK, Teerijoki-Oksa T, Virtanen A, et al. Sensory regeneration following intraoperatively verified trigeminal nerve injury. Neurology 2004;62(11): 1951–7.

42. Kehlet H, Jensen TS, Woolf CJ. Persistent postsurgical pain: risk factors and prevention. Lancet 2006;367(9522):1618–25.

43. Gregg JM. Surgical management of inferior alveolar nerve injuries (Part II): The case for delayed management. J Oral Maxillofac Surg 1995;53(11): 1330–3.

44. Robinson PP, Loescher AR, Smith KG. A prospective, quantitative study on the clinical outcome of lingual nerve repair. Br J Oral Maxillofac Surg 2000;38(4): 255–63.

45. Benoliel R, Kahn J, Eliav E. Peripheral painful traumatic trigeminal neuropathies. Oral Dis 2012;18(4): 317–32.

46. Haviv Y, Zadik Y, Sharav Y, et al. Painful traumatic trigeminal neuropathy: an open study on the pharmacotherapeutic response to stepped treatment. J Oral Facial Pain Headache 2014;28(1):52–60.

Soft Tissue Grafting Around Teeth and Implants

George R. Deeb, DDS, MD[a],*, Janina Golob Deeb, DDS, MS[b]

KEYWORDS

- Free gingival graft • Subepithelial connective tissue graft • Recession • Soft tissue defect • Allograft
- Xenograft

KEY POINTS

- Esthetic appearance and functional longevity for teeth and implants often requires conversion of unfavorable soft tissue traits to more favorable ones.
- Improvement of tissue quality and quantity can be accomplished with many different techniques and materials, and largely depends on clinical presentation of the case and the familiarity of the clinician with the procedures and materials available.
- Identification of causal factors, selection of appropriate surgical technique, and evidence-based material selection lead to predictable success when improving soft tissue characteristics around teeth or implants.

THE IDEAL CHARACTERISTICS OF THE SOFT TISSUE TOOTH/IMPLANT INTERFACE

The presence of healthy attached tissue at the tooth and implant soft tissue interface correlates with long-term success and stability in function and esthetics. Not only can a lack of keratinized tissue facilitate plaque aggregation around teeth and implants but it can also lead to recession of free soft tissue margin in the esthetic zone. The thicker periodontium is less prone to recession, because of the thickness of the cortical bone as well as the thickness of the surrounding gingiva.

Treatment of mucogingival deficiencies has become a large part of practices involving teeth and implants. The ramifications of not having an adequate keratinized tissue surrounding teeth have been studied extensively for decades,[1,2] and have also extended into implantology. The presence of gingiva is strongly correlated with optimal soft and hard tissue health.[3] However, in patients maintaining proper plaque control, the absence of attached gingiva around teeth does not result in an increased incidence of soft tissue recession.[1,4] It has been shown in long-term studies that even minimal amounts of keratinized tissue can provide long-term stability of soft tissue margin in the presence of good plaque control.[1]

Early studies suggested that the recession of soft tissue margin around implants may be the result of the remodeling of the periimplant soft tissue barrier. Lack of masticatory mucosa and the mobility of periimplant soft tissue were related to more pronounced soft tissue recession around implants.[5] Plaque-induced inflammation has been shown to cause recession when mucosal margins, rather than gingiva, are surrounding implants.[6] Thicker keratinized tissue facilitates plaque removal around implants. Plaque has been found as the causal factor in periodontal diseases[7] as

[a] Department of Oral and Maxillofacial Surgery, School of Dentistry, Virginia Commonwealth University, 521 North 11th Street, Richmond, VA 23298, USA; [b] Departments of Periodontics and General Practice, School of Dentistry, Virginia Commonwealth University, 521 North 11th Street, Richmond, VA 23298, USA
* Corresponding author.
E-mail address: gdeeb@vcu.edu

Oral Maxillofacial Surg Clin N Am 27 (2015) 425–448
http://dx.doi.org/10.1016/j.coms.2015.04.010
1042-3699/15/$ – see front matter © 2015 Elsevier Inc. All rights reserved.

well as periimplant inflammation, and its removal is paramount in tooth and implant long-term health.

Facilitating plaque removal is not the only indication when considering improvement of soft tissue structure surrounding teeth or implants. Esthetic demands for implants have become as high as those for natural dentition. Exposed metal or any visible discrepancies in soft tissue volume or margins suggesting an implant-supported prosthesis in anterior regions have become largely unacceptable by patients. Implant-supported restorations and teeth restored side by side should be in harmony, not only when it comes to prosthetic suprastructures but also in levels of gingival margins, thickness, color, and contour of adjacent gingiva.

Several soft tissue grafting procedures has been developed to improve both the volume of keratinized tissue and the soft tissue contour around implants. Concepts for these surgical techniques have been drawn from procedures developed to enhance soft tissue support around teeth.

DEVELOPMENT OF MUCOGINGIVAL DIAGNOSIS AND SURGERY

The term mucogingival surgery was first introduced by Friedman[8] in 1957 in reference to correcting relationships between mucosa and gingiva around teeth. In the following decades, that term has expanded to include numerous procedures used to correct and alter defects, position, thickness, and the width of keratinized tissue surrounding teeth. As implantology has expanded and esthetic demand for prosthetic replacements has grown, periodontal plastic surgery procedures have been developed around implants and edentulous ridges restored with pontics and removable prostheses. The term periodontal plastic surgery was introduced by Miller[9] in 1988 and presently includes procedures to prevent or correct oral soft tissue defects of anatomic, developmental, traumatic, and disease-related origin.

GINGIVAL RECESSION AROUND TEETH AND IMPLANTS

The displacement of the soft tissue margin in an apical direction from the cementoenamel junction leads to exposure of the root surface of a tooth, and is referred to as a marginal soft tissue recession.[10] When the soft tissue margin recedes apically around an implant, it can lead to exposure of the abutment or implant body depending on the extent of displacement, as well as the design of the implant and its suprastructure. In both cases, the term soft tissue margin is inclusive of either mucosa or gingiva, whichever is present at the site.

When considering correction of recession it is important to identify the presence and the amount of gingiva as well as causal factors contributing to displacement of soft tissue margin. Causal factors of soft tissue recession around teeth include the quantity and quality of surrounding keratinized attached tissue, supporting alveolar bone, and the level of plaque control of the affected area. Causes of soft tissue defects surrounding implants include poor implant spatial positioning, incorrect abutment contour, excessive implant diameter, horizontal biologic width formation, and periodontal phenotype.[11]

CLASSIFICATION OF RECESSION

Several classification systems have been developed to assess and quantify the amount of surrounding soft tissue and osseous components.

Sullivan and Atkins[12] introduced a classification system in 1968 to describe recession around teeth. This classification system was based on the width and length of recession. It was already established at that time that those parameters determined the amount of root coverage obtainable with soft tissue grafting procedures.

Miller[13] introduced his classification system in 1985 (**Box 1**). He related the extent of the soft tissue recession to the location of the mucogingival junction as well as the height of interproximal clinical attachment adjacent to the surface affected by the recession.

Miller's[13] classification is a helpful diagnostic tool in treatment planning and setting realistic expectations for both patients and clinicians. Root coverage can be predictably obtained in class I and II groups, only partially in class III, and not at all in class IV. Properly diagnosing the soft tissue recession is helpful in choosing a proper soft tissue grafting technique and setting expectations for surgical outcome.

In 1999, the International Workshop for Classification of Periodontal Diseases and Conditions formed by the American Academy of Periodontology agreed on a new classification system for periodontal diseases. Category VIII on developmental or acquired deformities and conditions was added to provide more comprehensive diagnostic tool for soft tissue characteristics around teeth and edentulous ridges (**Table 1**).[14]

ESTHETIC CONSIDERATIONS

Loss of gingival symmetry is most notable on anterior teeth[15] and implants, especially with regard to the principles of gingival zenith positions and levels.

Box 1
Miller classification system of marginal soft tissue recession

Class I:

- Recession does not extend to mucogingival junction
- There is no loss of interproximal clinical attachment

Class II:

- Recession extends to or beyond mucogingival junction
- There is no loss of interproximal clinical attachment

Class III:

- Recession extends to or beyond mucogingival junction
- Some interproximal clinical attachment loss is present or malpositioning of teeth is present

Class IV:

- Recession extends to or beyond mucogingival junction
- Severe interproximal clinical attachment loss is present or severe malpositioning of teeth is present

From Miller PD. A classification of marginal tissue recession. Int J Periodontics Restorative Dent 1985;5:9.

Tarnow showed that the gingival zenith line of the lateral incisors relative to the adjacent central incisor and canine teeth is positioned more coronally by approximately 1 mm. These reference points should be used as guides to reestablish the proper intratooth gingival zenith line of the maxillary anterior teeth during root coverage and reconstructive procedures.[16]

THICK VERSUS THIN GINGIVAL ARCHITECTURE

Treatment planning for dental implant placement should consist of assessment of the periodontal biotype of both the proposed implant site and the adjacent dentition. This soft tissue assessment is particularly important for the immediate implant case as well as treatment in the esthetic zone (**Fig. 1**).

The thick, flat periodontal biotype is characterized by dense fibrotic gingiva. There is a larger zone of attached gingiva, with smaller embrasures associated with square-shaped teeth. Gingival scallop on anterior teeth is flat and does not exceed 3 to 4 mm. The contact points are long and are located in the middle third of the teeth. Soft tissue is supported by thick bone, with the high incidence of exostosis resisting the tendency for recession to occur.

The thin periodontal biotype displays a thin, scalloped gingiva with a narrow zone of attachment. The teeth are triangular and have long interproximal contacts in the incisal third region. Gingival scallop on anterior teeth can reach 4 to 6 mm. The thin periodontium often reveals undulating contours of the prominent roots of the teeth alternating with the concave interdental bone. In this biotype, bone is thin and has a high incidence of dehiscence and fenestration defects. Brushing can result in soft tissue recession over the

Table 1
Developmental or acquired deformities and conditions

Mucogingival Deformities and Conditions Around Teeth	Mucogingival Deformities and Conditions on Edentulous Ridges

1. Gingival/soft tissue recession
  a. Facial or lingual surfaces
  b. Interproximal (papillary)
	1. Vertical and/or horizontal ridge deficiency

2. Lack of keratinized gingiva	2. Lack of gingiva/keratinized tissue
3. Decreased vestibular depth	3. Gingival/soft tissue enlargement
4. Aberrant frenum/muscle position	4. Aberrant frenum/muscle position

5. Gingival excess
  a. Pseudopocket
  b. Inconsistent gingival margin
  c. Excessive gingival display
  d. Gingival enlargement
	5. Decreased vestibular depth

6. Abnormal color	6. Abnormal color

From Armitage GC. Development of a classification system for periodontal diseases and conditions. Ann Periodontol 1999;4(1):1–6.

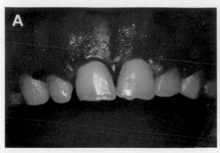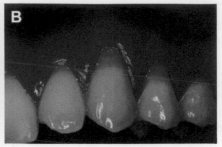

Fig. 1. (*A*) Thick, flat periodontal biotype is characterized by dense fibrotic gingiva, large zone of attached gingiva, smaller embrasures, and square-shaped teeth. (*B*) Thin periodontal biotype has a thin, scalloped gingiva with a narrow zone of attachment. The teeth are triangular, and the thin periodontium often reveals undulating contours of the prominent roots of the teeth and bone.

dehiscence defects, which continues until the bone margin is reached.

Kan and colleagues[17] evaluated the dimensions of the periimplant mucosa around 2-stage maxillary anterior single implants. The investigators concluded that the level of the interproximal papilla around the implant is independent of the proximal bone level next to the implant, but is related to the interproximal bone level next to the adjacent tooth. Greater periimplant mucosal dimensions were noted in the presence of a thick periimplant biotype compared with a thin biotype.

THE RELATIONSHIP BETWEEN IMPLANT PLACEMENT AND SOFT TISSUE

The relationship between the bone and soft tissue ultimately defines the final esthetic result. The three-dimensional relationship between the implant and surrounding bone determines the soft tissue contours and interdental papilla.

Implants Should Be Placed 3 mm Below the Facial Gingival Margin in an Apicocoronal Dimension for the Following Reasons

- To allow for prosthetic abutment placement and formation of biologic width.
- To allow for creation of a natural emergence profile.
- To allow for restorative margins to be placed subgingivally.
- To allow for age-related recession without immediate exposure of the implant abutment interface.

Implants Should Be Placed in a Buccolingual Dimension 1 to 2 mm Palatal from the Anticipated Facial Margin of the Restoration

Schneider and colleagues[18] recommend a 2-mm palatal placement in anticipation of a 1.4-mm lateral bone loss as a guideline.

Kan and colleagues[17] recommend that the placement be 1 mm palatal in relation to the facial emergence profiles of the adjacent teeth, and not less than 1 mm because of the risk of losing the facial bone and soft tissue.

The Implant Should Be Placed with the Platform at the Level of the Gingival Zenith and 3 mm Apical to the Soft Tissue Margin

Gingival zenith position (GZP) does not line up with the middle of the facial surface of the tooth or vertical bisected midline (VBM) for all anterior tooth groups. The largest discrepancy between GZP and VBM was noted in maxillary central incisors with GZP located 1 mm distal to the VBM.[16] The lateral incisors showed an average of 0.4 mm discrepancy, whereas the canines showed almost no deviations of the GZP from the VBM.[16]

Implants Should Be Placed with a Minimum of 1.5 mm Between the Adjacent Tooth and Implant

Esposito and colleagues[19] indicated a strong correlation between bone loss of adjacent teeth and horizontal distance of the implant fixture to the tooth. The greatest amount of bone loss was noted at the lateral incisor position.

Implants Should Be Placed with an Interimplant Distance of at Least 3 mm in a 2-Stage Protocol

Tarnow and colleagues[20] in their retrospective study of patients with 2 adjacent implants found that when implants were placed within 3 mm of each other they developed 1.04 mm of interproximal bone loss compared with implants placed with greater than 3.0 mm of bone between them, which lost only 0.45 mm of bone. The loss of height of interproximal bone has an effect on papilla support.

PAPILLA

Maintaining papillae between anterior teeth leads to optimal gingival contour and appearance. Surgical techniques for soft tissue grafting around teeth all include papilla preservation in height and at least partial thickness.

Papilla Adjacent to Teeth

Maintenance of interproximal papillae is more predictable in periodontally healthy patients because of predictable tissue rebound over time, which can be anticipated by the height of interproximal bone on the adjacent teeth.[21] Complete papilla fill has been observed when the distance from the contact point to the bone crest was 5 mm or less. When the distance exceeds 6 mm, papillae are present only 56% of time.[22] Restorative solutions for manipulation of contact point location are used to reduce the distance from contact point to the crest as well as adding the length to the contact surface and bulk to coronal contours. Surgical techniques intended to increase the volume of papillae include case reports of the use of platelet-rich fibrin,[23] injection of hyaluronic acid–based gel,[24] and connective tissue graft with coronally advanced flap (CAF).[25] Most case reports on these techniques represent a small number of cases and short-term follow-up, failing to show long-term stability.

Papillae Adjacent to Implants

The projected height of a papilla next to an implant largely depends on whether it is adjacent to the tooth or another implant. Tarnow and colleagues[26] observed that, when placing 2 implants adjacent to each other, only an average of 3.4 mm of soft tissue height can be expected to form over the interimplant crest of bone.

Schropp and Isidor[27] evaluated soft tissue levels and papilla dimensions for early versus delayed single implants. Implants placed 10 days following extraction tended to be superior to delayed implants regarding soft tissue appearance at crown delivery as well as 10 years later. The implant region does not seem to influence the papilla, although patients younger than 50 years received significantly better papilla scores. An apically located bone level at the tooth neighboring the implant negatively influenced the papilla dimension. In contrast, the presence of a bone defect buccally to the implant at second-stage surgery did not have a negative impact on the gingival margin 10 years after implant placement.[27]

Provisional Restoration

The selection of the provisional restoration significantly influences healing of the soft tissues (**Fig. 2**). Placement of an immediate provisional affects the periimplant tissue morphology according to its emergence profile.[28] Papilla preservation as well as restoration can be accomplished. Part of the anterior esthetic case planning should involve planning for the provisional restoration. In general, fixed provisionals work better than removable provisionals. Screw-retained provisional restorations are preferred in cases in which soft tissue contours

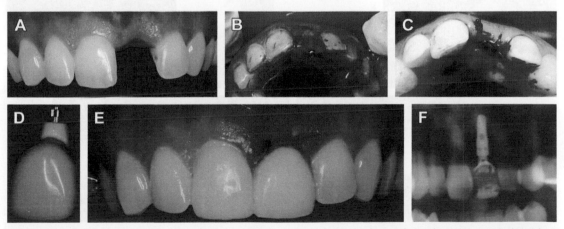

Fig. 2. (*A*) Preoperative view of a #9 edentulous ridge planned for a single-tooth implant. (*B*) Surgical guide in place during implant placement. Note that the guide pin is palatal in order maintain the buccal plate and prevent recession of the soft tissue. (*C*) Intraoperative view with a 3.0-mm healing abutment in place. The 3.0-mm healing abutment is flush with the gingiva and ensures that proper emergence can be achieved. (*D*) Screw-retained provisional with the correct gingival contours. (*E*) The provisional restoration in place along with the veneer showing acceptable esthetic outcome. (*F*) Postoperative panoramic film showing the implant and provisional crown in place.

are critical. Screw-retained restorations avoid cement-caused periimplant inflammation. Screw-retained restorations also allow retrieval and adjustment of the contours of the restoration, which are critical in guiding papilla restoration. Contact points on adjacent teeth as well as emergence dictate the final result.

SOFT TISSUE MANAGEMENT BEFORE IMPLANT PLACEMENT
Extraction Sockets

In the absence of keratinized tissue or when gingiva is present but inflamed and fragile, it is important to incorporate procedures to preserve and augment surrounding connective tissue in early phases of treatment (**Fig. 3**A–H). Following extraction in an anterior segment with deficient gingiva, the clinician might choose not to proceed with an immediate implant placement but rather resort to a staged approach.

When performing the socket preservation procedure, anatomic features of the socket which will become a future implant site should be assessed and improved with grafting techniques. Closure after extraction can be manipulated in ways to create or move keratinized tissue for future implant placement. Covering bone graft with a membrane or soft tissue graft results in expansion of gingival tissue. Obtaining primary closure by advancing the flap often comes at the expense of displacing or losing facial keratinized tissue.

Patient factors that define the success of an implant placement include bone level, buccal bone thickness, soft and hard tissue relationship, and gingival biotype.[29]

Bone grafting for socket preservation or ridge augmentation techniques can be implemented to improve osseous characteristics of the site. The bone support will define the soft tissue architecture after healing. Connective tissue grafts or pedicle grafts can be used to augment deficient

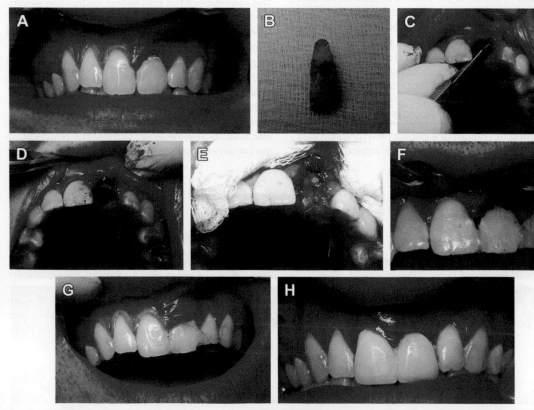

Fig. 3. (A) Preoperative view of a patient with a thin, scalloped periodontium with external resorption of tooth #9. (B) Extracted tooth with external resorption visible on the buccal aspect of the tooth. (C) Postextraction view showing buccal wall defect. (D) Rigid collagen membrane bridging the buccal wall dehiscence before placement of bone graft into the socket. The connective tissue graft for socket coverage has been harvested. (E) Connective tissue graft sutured into place over the socket preservation procedure. (F) Natural tooth bonded into place postoperatively and without contacting the ridge. (G) One-week postoperative view showing improved bulk and color after socket preservation procedure. (H) Four-month postoperative result.

soft tissue components. Autogenous grafts can be allowed to heal in part by secondary intention further enhancing the amount of keratinized tissue available for future implant placement.

Note that immediate implant placement into sockets with deficient facial keratinized tissue and thin buccal bone may lead to unpredictable height and contour of soft tissue margin and esthetic outcome. Delaying implant placement and creating healthy and adequate amounts of gingiva first yields more predictable esthetic results.

SOFT TISSUE MANAGEMENT AT THE TIME OF IMPLANT PLACEMENT

Sites augmented with subepithelial connective tissue grafts (SCTG) at the time of implant placement have better esthetics and thicker periimplant tissues.[30] When SCTG is used with immediate implant placement and provisionalization in the esthetic zone it significantly improves maintenance of facial gingival level.[31]

Grunder[32] measured the dimension of the labial volume before and 6 months after implant placement in the maxillary anterior area with or without SCTG using a flapless tunnel technique. The nongrafted group had an average 1.063-mm loss of volume, whereas the grafted group presented with a slight gain of 0.34 mm. These results confirmed the effectiveness of placing a soft tissue graft at the time of immediate implant placement in the esthetic zone.[32]

In totally edentulous patient, firm keratinized tissue surrounding the implants and adequate vestibular depth are among the determining factors for long-term implant success. In the staged approach of mandibular implant reconstruction, adequate vestibular depth and gingiva surrounding the implants can be readily established at the time of implant placement or when the implants are uncovered.

However, in cases in which extractions and alveolar ridge reduction are done in the mandible immediately before implant placement, surgeons have a challenging task to maintain adequate keratinized tissue and vestibular depth on buccal and lingual aspects of the implants. Securing both flaps apically to a fixed and stable bony anchorage greatly reduces the likelihood of prolapse of the buccal vestibule and elevation of the lingual floor into prosthetic space as well as beyond the implant margins. This fixed anchorage is especially important in patients who cannot wear prosthetic devices during the healing phase.[33] Single-stage surgery with the placement of healing abutments allows the patient the additional benefit

of greater prosthesis retention during the healing stage (**Fig. 4**).

Treatment Planning for Soft Tissue Grafting Around Teeth and Implants

The ultimate goal of soft tissue grafting is to improve the prognosis of affected teeth or implants. Prognosis depends on the ability to practice good plaque control and to maintain healthy soft tissue margins. In esthetic areas, achieving optimal soft tissue contours around teeth, implants, or prostheses is also of great importance.

Numerous techniques involving soft tissue manipulation from adjacent or distant donor sites have been developed to cover exposed roots and enhance soft tissue structure in areas with deficient or absent gingiva. Conventional periodontal plastic surgical techniques are generally separated into pedicle grafts and free soft tissue grafts (**Box 2**).

FREE SOFT TISSUE GRAFTING

When treatment planning a soft tissue graft it is important to consider the goal. Indications can be driven by esthetic demands with the purpose of establishing a harmony with regard to health, height, volume, color, and contours of gingiva with the surrounding dentition.

In addition, indications are often related to inability to remove plaque efficiently around teeth and implants surrounded by thin mucosa, resulting in recession. Longitudinal evaluations conclude that minimizing inflammation is sufficient and is necessary to maintain attachment levels despite the width of keratinized tissue surrounding teeth.[34] Therefore it is important to educate patients about how to properly exercise oral hygiene and to consider soft tissue surgery in appropriate circumstances when enhanced soft tissue will result in an improved prognosis of the grafted tooth or implant.

In cases in which the sole goal is to increase the amount of keratinized tissue, the most suitable technique remains a free gingival graft. When the desired outcome includes coverage of exposed root, connective tissue grafting provides more predictable outcomes.[35]

THE FREE GINGIVAL GRAFT

The term free gingival graft was introduced in 1966 by Nabers[36] and this graft is now referred to as free epithelialized soft tissue graft. This technique originally used tissue removed after gingivectomy, but was later modified to include palatal or masticatory gingiva as a primary donor source.[37]

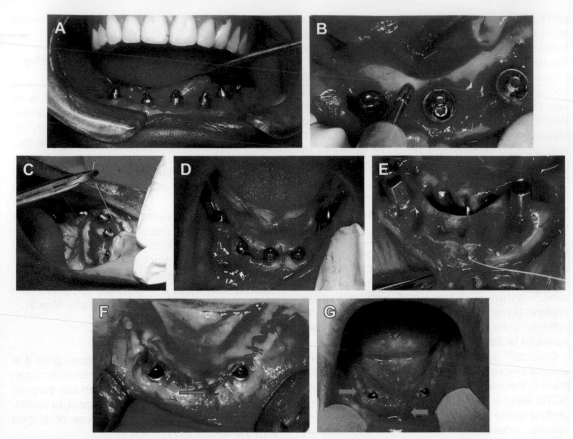

Fig. 4. (*A*) Five lower implants placed for an immediate loaded full-arch provisional restoration. (*B*) Close-up view of a fissure burr being used to make an interimplant osteotomy of the lingual cortical bone as a means of stabilizing flaps in an apical position. In this example the lingual cortex is being perforated because of the wide buccolingual dimension of the alveolar ridge as well as to avoid inadvertent damage to the implants. (*C*) Intraoperative view showing the suturing sequence. The operator passes from the buccal tissues through the alveolus and through the lingual tissues before tying the knot over the ridge to secure the tissues. (*D*) Intraoperative view with 3 transalveolar sutures in place. The sutures are placed in the interimplant bone and secured. The rest of the final closure is completed in chromic gut suture. Note the preservation of keratinized tissue and apical position of the flaps. (*E*) Intraoperative view after implantation showing the needle being passed through the alveolus in order to show the placement of the transalveolar osteotomy in a 5-mm apical position. For altering vestibular height the osteotomy should be placed apically, as shown. For use the buccal flap should be engaged before entering the osteotomy and the lingual flap on exiting, as in **Fig. 3**. (*F*) Immediate postoperative view of the closure using the transalveolar suture (*arrow*) securing the flaps in an apical position in order to increase vestibular depth. (*G*) One week after surgery showing favorable healing and stable tissue adaptation around the implants. The transalveolar sutures (*arrows*) are still intact.

The autogenous free gingival graft can be subdivided by thickness of the donor tissue into 3 categories:

1. Thin (0.5–0.8 mm)
2. Average (0.9–1.4 mm)
3. Thick (1.5 to >2 mm)

The thin graft is well suited to increasing the amount of keratinized gingiva and provides the best color match. A thin graft has to be placed in intimate contact with an intact blood supply of the recipient site with the incision on the recipient site placed submarginally. Placement over an exposed root surface should be avoided because

it is not suited when root coverage is attempted. The thin free gingival graft heals the fastest but also has the highest percentage of secondary shrinkage after healing (25%–30%).[38,39] The donor site is shallow and therefore heals mostly uneventfully.

The average-thickness graft is best suited for all types of grafting except root coverage. This graft provides acceptable appearance and better protection against future recession than the thin graft. The donor site is deeper, which can cause more complications following surgery. A palatal stent is recommended to protect the donor site and ensure blood clot stabilization.

<table>
<tr><td>

Box 2
Conventional periodontal plastic surgical techniques

Pedicle graft

Flap advancement procedures:

- Coronally positioned flaps
- Semilunar coronally positioned flaps

Flap rotation procedures:

- Laterally sliding flap
- Partial-thickness double pedicle graft
- Rotational flap
- Transpositioned flap

Free soft tissue grafts

- Free gingival grafts
- SCTGs

Free soft tissue grafts can be further divided depending on the source of origin into:

- Autogenous grafts
- Allografts
- Xenografts

</td></tr>
</table>

The thick free gingival graft can be used for covering exposed root surfaces.[40] When root coverage is desired, a 1.25-mm or thicker graft should be used. Recipient bed margins should include epithelial denudation of marginal and papillary gingiva.

The thick graft undergoes greater primary contraction, but the secondary contraction is minimal because of thick lamina propria. Thick grafts are more resistant to future recession. There tends to be an increase in root coverage over a 1-year period following surgery, known as creeping attachment, which is most often observed with thick grafts.[41] Once healed, thick grafts result in less esthetically acceptable appearance because of color and thickness incompatibility with adjacent gingiva (**Fig. 5**).

Indications for Free Gingival Graft

Free gingival grafts remain the gold standard for augmentation of width and thickness of keratinized tissue around teeth and implants. It has remained a predictable technique when objectives include:

- Augmentation of gingival dimensions
- Elimination of the frenum
- Increase of vestibular depth
- Improvement of local anatomic factors associated with facial tooth position
- Large, prominent roots with dehiscence
- Stabilization of progressive gingival recession
- Correction of ridge deformities and undercuts
- Protection of denture bearing surface[42]

Free gingival grafting can be used as a 2-stage procedure for root coverage with coronal advancement once the graft has healed. It has also been found to achieve root coverage as a 1-step surgical procedure in 44%[43,44] and up to 89.9% of the sites when applied appropriately.[40]

Despite its ability to obtain root coverage, free gingival graft is not suitable for areas with esthetic concerns. Previous studies have shown that free gingiva grafted onto ectopic oral sites retains the tissue characteristics of their donor site, which may affect the esthetics of the grafted site.[45,46]

Technique

The incision is made at the mucogingival junction along the length of recipient area and extended to adjacent teeth; however, it should not involve the sulci of the nongrafted adjacent teeth. On the mesial and distal aspects, the horizontal incision is connected to 2 vertical incisions at 90° or slightly divergent toward mucosa. A split-thickness dissection is performed, leaving in place periosteum and deepening the fornix. Preparation of

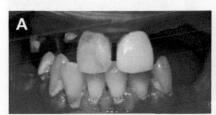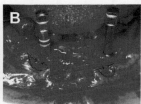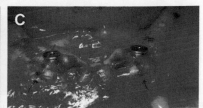

Fig. 5. (*A*) Preoperative view of a patient presenting for a 2-implant overdenture with a thin periodontium and recession. (*B*) Intraoperative view after implant placement. The blue lines will be deepithelialized and closed in a double papilla fashion (*arrows*) in order to increase the keratinized tissue. (*C*) The final closure over the connective tissue grafts. The arrows indicate the double papilla closure. These grafts increase keratinized tissue and convert the patient to a thicker periodontal biotype.

the recipient bed should extend 3 mm past the edge of the denuded root surface and include removal of aberrant frenum.

When root coverage is also the objective of the procedure, the initial horizontal incision should be placed at the level of the desired new gingival level. The level of gingiva anticipated following grafting can be either at the cemento-enamel junction for Miller class I and II recession defects or below it for class III and IV. The larger donor tissue is easier to stabilize, therefore rendering root coverage more successful. Thick grafts that cover only 1 tooth are harder to suture and stabilize, making them less predictable for use in root coverage procedures.

Gingival grafts should be excised from the donor site with recipient site size and shape in mind and contoured to the recipient area.[36]

Suturing the graft to the recipient site should completely immobilize the graft to encourage the anastomosing of capillaries by maintaining intimate contact with the recipient site vascular bed. The thicker grafts should be slightly stretched to keep capillaries open, thus enabling the establishment of the blood supply to the graft. Interrupted sutures are used on the edges. Sling sutures around grafted teeth ensure intimate contact of the graft interproximally and elimination of the dead space between graft and recipient bed.

At present, free gingival grafts are not used as often as in the past because of less than optimal esthetics and a more uncomfortable postoperative course than newer subepithelial techniques.

SOFT TISSUE GRAFTING ON IMPLANTS VERSUS TEETH

Free gingival grafting provides a wider zone of keratinized tissue and promotes a tight adaptation of denser tissue around implants, which allows better plaque control and gingival health. Only a small number of studies are available reporting long-term stability of exposed implant coverage compared with studies performed on teeth. From available data, it is suggestive that gained soft tissue coverage on teeth remains stable in the long term compared with implants (**Figs. 6** and **7**).

The technique used by Burkhardt and colleagues[47] to cover approximately 3 mm of soft tissue recession on buccal aspect of implants resembles in every step techniques used to cover exposed root surfaces with SCTG on teeth. However, despite achieving immediate recession coverage of more than 100% following surgery, that gain was not maintained and shrank to 66% at the 6-month follow-up. In contrast, similar soft tissue defects on implants were treated by Zucchelli and colleagues[48] also using connective tissue grafts. At 1 year they observed a mean coverage of 96% and a significant increase in the amount of keratinized tissue. The main difference between the two studies was the removal of the crown and reshaping and polishing of the implant abutment before surgery, allowing better adaptation between the graft and abutment. Reshaping and polishing the implant abutment closely resembles the way grafting is performed over

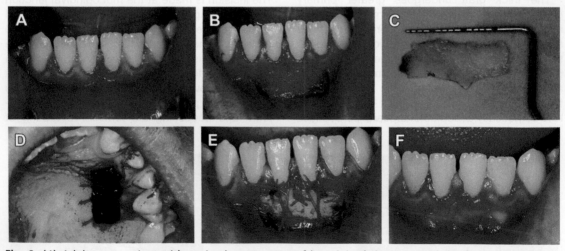

Fig. 6. (*A*) Adolescent patient with an inadequate zone of keratinized tissue around the facial aspect of the mandibular incisors. (*B*) Split-thickness dissection of the anterior mandible to prepare the recipient bed for palatal free gingival grafting. Note that the flap has been positioned apically in order to avoid coronal migration. (*C*) Free gingival graft harvested from the palate. (*D*) Palatal donor site with Surgicel and Periacryl dressing oversewn with chromic gut suture. (*E*) Palatal graft sutured into place using chromic gut suture. (*F*) One week after surgery showing an increased zone of attached tissue.

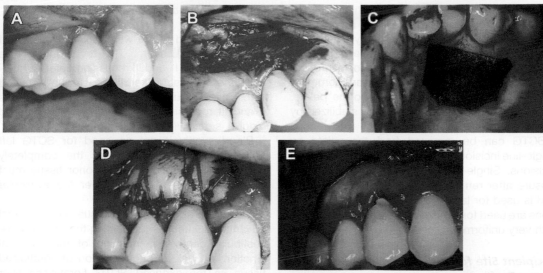

Fig. 7. (*A*) A single-tooth implant showing a lack of keratinized tissue. (*B*) Supraperiosteal dissection in preparation for the free gingival graft. (*C*) A template in place before graft harvest. (*D*) The free gingival graft secured into the recipient bed. (*E*) The final result showing increased keratinized tissue. Coverage of the porcelain at the apical portion of the restoration was not achieved (and rarely is).

root surfaces with root planning, reshaping, conditioning, and placement of grafts in close proximity to recipient surfaces. Addition of abutment and crown modifications provides more space and better adaptation of the graft into the recipient site. Provisional crowns can be modified to guide and sculpt soft tissue during healing.[49]

SUBEPITHELIAL CONNECTIVE TISSUE GRAFT

This technique is currently used in most soft tissue grafts performed in periodontal plastic surgery. The connective tissue graft, also known as SCTG was introduced in 1980 by Langer and Calagna.[50] Its use was described for root coverage and ridge augmentation procedures.

The donor site was the patient's palate, the graft was 1 to 2 mm thick, and split-thickness recipient bed preparation was suggested to provide double blood supply to the newly added tissue graft.[50]

The autogenous SCTG is divided by thickness of the donor tissue into 3 categories:

1. Thin (0.5–0.8 mm)
2. Average (0.9–1.4 mm)
3. Thick (1.5 to >2 mm)

The thickness of the graft proved to have an effect on the amount of shrinkage and the rate of healing of the graft that occurred following surgery. Rapid revascularization can be expected when uniform thin or intermediate grafts are placed on a periosteal recipient site. An uneven, thick graft placed on a site of denuded bone favored a prolonged period of revascularization and delayed healing.[51]

Technique for Subepithelial Connective Tissue Graft

Donor site for subepithelial connective tissue graft

Masticatory mucosa on the palate between palatal raphae and maxillary posterior teeth is the most common location for the donor site for SCTG (see **Fig. 16**). It is composed of connective tissue and loosely organized glandular and adipose tissue.[52] The best-quality connective tissue is found closest to the teeth; however, harvesting tissue closer than 2 mm to the teeth places those teeth at risk for developing postoperative gingival recession caused by inadequate blood supply to the apex of the retained flap.

Surgeons harvesting SCTG from the palate must be familiar with the anatomy and characteristics of this donor site. It is important to avoid the nerves and vessels located in the greater palatine groove at the junction of vertical and horizontal palate. The palatal vault height varies from 7 mm to 17 mm, with an average distance of 12 mm from the neurovascular line.

The incision is started 2 mm from the soft tissue margin on the palatal aspect of the teeth and it should end 2 mm above the neurovascular line. The width of donor tissue can therefore vary from 3 to 13 mm, with an average width of 8 mm.

The size of SCTG needed depends on the demands of the recipient site; however, for most sites, 5 to 9 mm is an adequate width. Limitations that the shallow vault represents as a donor site should be considered before surgery. Alternative sources for donor tissue are available and should be used in such cases. Encroaching on neurovascular structures can lead to bleeding and some degree of postoperative paresthesia to the palate. Donor sites can often be adequately stabilized by suturing (**Figs. 11**C and **16**C).

SCTG can be removed from the palate by single-line incision (see **Fig. 16**B) or double parallel incisions. Single-line incision allows for primary closure after removal of the graft (see **Fig. 16**C) and is used for larger grafts. Double parallel incisions are used for smaller grafts and provide grafts with very uniform thickness.

Recipient Site for Subepithelial Connective Tissue Graft

Modifications of preparation of the recipient site have followed the introduction of the original technique. To eliminate vertical incisions, envelope flaps were explored for recipient sites with similar success.[53] Connective tissue grafts are used in combination with many different recipient site pedicle flap designs. SCTG can be either completely covered or left partially exposed. Harris and colleagues[54] compared 3 variations of recipient site flap design in conjunction with connective tissue graft. Techniques including coronally positioned flap, double pedicle flap, and a tunneling procedure over an autogenous connective tissue graft were all effective in obtaining root coverage and improving clinical parameters.

Partially covered subepithelial connective tissue graft

Partially covered SCTG was originally described by Langer and Langer.[55] This technique can be used for class I, II, and III recession defects; however, the increase in keratinized tissue obtained with this technique makes it more suitable for class II and III recession defects in which keratinized gingiva is deficient (**Fig. 8**).

Blood supply is not as good for SCTG left partially exposed as it is for the completely covered SCTG, therefore the donor tissue must be thick enough to survive over the avascular root of the tooth.

Partial graft coverage techniques offer several advantages, such as maintaining the preoperative vestibular depth and position of mucogingival junction, as well as augmentation of keratinized tissue as the exposed SCTG keratinizes over when left exposed.[56] Submerged grafts without epithelial collar performed better esthetically, whereas exposed epithelial collar grafts resulted in better gingival augmentation with similar results in root coverage.[57] In spite of attempts to remove the epithelium, it remains in 80% of the grafts.[58]

Completely covered subepithelial connective tissue graft

Connective tissue grafts can be completely covered by the use of CAF. Vertical incisions can be used for increased access and to facilitate coronal repositioning; however, they decrease blood supply and can cause scarring.

In the absence of keratinized tissue before grafting, the flap to cover the graft consists of only

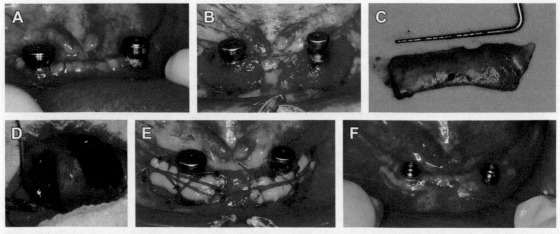

Fig. 8. (*A*) Preoperative clinical view showing 2 dental implants with inadequate keratinized tissue on the facial aspect. (*B*) Supraperiosteal dissection to prepare a bed for free gingival grafting. The apical flap margin is sutured to periosteum to prevent coronal migration during healing. (*C*) Palatal free gingival graft harvest. (*D*) Palatal donor sites. These sites can be dressed with Surgicel and Periacryl. (*E*) Free gingival grafts sutured into place using 3.0 chromic gut. (*F*) Eight weeks after surgery showing increased keratinized tissue.

mucosa. When covering an SCTG with a flap lacking keratinized tissue, the outer surface over the graft heals as nonkeratinized mucosa for a soft tissue margin. To alter the surface of a new soft tissue margin from mucosa to keratinized tissue once the graft has established its own blood supply, overlying mucosa can be released and apically positioned leaving SCTG exposed to keratinize over.

PARTIAL-THICKNESS DOUBLE PEDICLE GRAFT

The use of a double pedicle flap should be considered when the objective of grafting includes the increase of keratinized tissue. The overlying double pedicle slides laterally interproximal papillary keratinized tissue over the grafted root surface and, compared with a coronally positioned pedicle flap deficient in keratinized tissue, results in a larger increase of keratinized tissue (3.0 mm vs 1.8 mm) (**Fig. 9**).[59]

TECHNIQUE FOR PEDICLE FLAP WITH VERTICAL INCISIONS

The horizontal incision is made at the desired level of the future gingival margin, usually at the level of the CEJ. The incision extends to the interdental area adjacent to the terminal grafted tooth. When the second incision is used parallel to the first incision, it should be spaced as far apically from the first one as the recession measures on the exposed root. These incisions are then connected with mesial and distal vertical incisions that extend beyond the mucogingival junction to allow manipulation of the flap in the coronal direction. The recipient bed is prepared with split-thickness dissection to free the flap from the periosteum.

SCTG is sutured in place, extending to the edges of the recipient bed (**Fig. 10**B). The flap is then coronally advanced for as many millimeters as the recession measured before grafting (see **Fig. 10**).

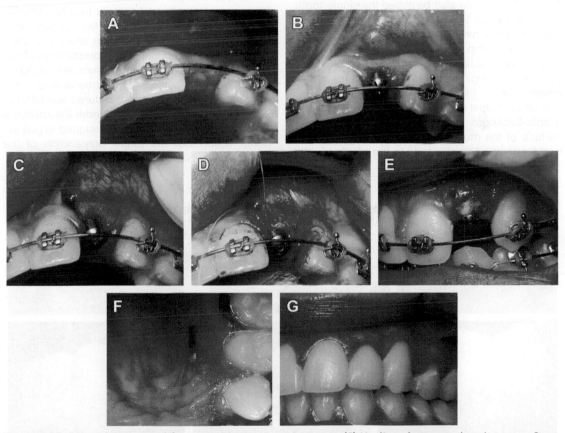

Fig. 9. (*A*) Punch technique used for uncovering at stage 2 surgery. (*B*) Healing abutment placed at stage 2 surgery. Note the horizontal ridge deficiency and narrow zone of attached tissue. (*C*) Papilla-sparing incision with vertical releases is being elevated in preparation for connective tissue grafting to buccally augment the zone of attachment. (*D*) Palatal connective tissue graft being sutured in place. (*E*) One week after surgery showing buccal and vertical augmentation of the site. (*F*) The connective tissue donor site 1 week after surgery. (*G*) Final restoration at 1 year after surgery showing improved buccal and vertical soft tissue contours.

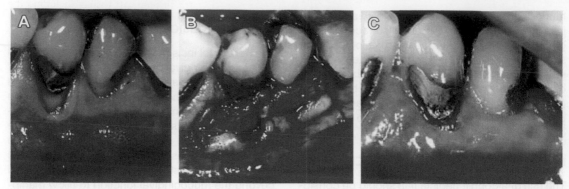

Fig. 10. Connective tissue graft and pedicle flap (*A*) Preoperative view of lower left premolar area. Note receding soft tissue margin with minimal amount of keratinized tissue present on tooth #21 and amalgam restoration extending onto root surface. (*B*) Intraoperative view showing recipient site with pedicle flap and SCTG sutured to obtain desired root coverage apically of amalgam restoration. (*C*) Four weeks postoperatively, teeth #20 and #21 present with improved soft tissue support and good root coverage apically of margins of preexisting restorations.

TECHNIQUE FOR ENVELOPE FLAP

This technique can also be called the single-tooth tunnel or pouch technique. The SCTG is sutured into a recipient tunnel donor site without reflecting a traditional flap. The envelope flap maintains ample blood supply from the adjacent papillary, overlying mucogingival and underlying mucoperiosteal sides.

A small scalpel blade is placed in the sulcus and a split-thickness pouch is developed under the surface of the mucogingival tissue. The recipient bed preparation must extend to the papilla slightly coronally to the CEJ. Papillary tissue is undermined but not reflected. The pouch must extend far enough laterally and apically to allow passive placement of the SCTG. Dissection for this technique is more difficult and tactile sensation is the only method of negotiating the preparation of the recipient site between periosteum and mucosa or gingiva. The suturing technique is also more challenging; however, fewer sutures are needed because of good graft stability under the envelope flap. The suturing technique is designed to pull the donor tissue into the tunnel preparation of the recipient site (See **Fig. 11**).

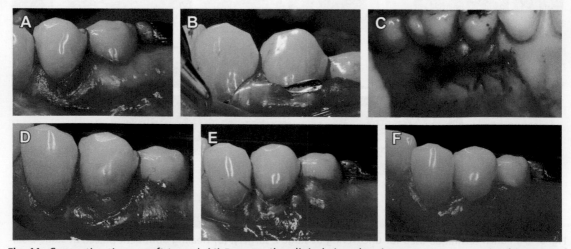

Fig. 11. Connective tissue graft tunnel. (*A*) Preoperative clinical view showing root exposure and a thin zone of keratinized tissue. (*B*) Subepithelial tunnel being prepared in a split-thickness dissection to receive the connective tissue. (*C*) Single-incision technique used to harvest the connective tissue graft. (*D*) Connective tissue graft placed into the subepithelial pocket. (*E*) Connective tissue graft and buccal flap sutured to the level of the CEJ. (*F*) One-month postoperative visit showing root coverage as well as an increased zone of keratinized tissue.

SEMILUNAR AND LATERAL SLIDING FLAPS

Semilunar coronally positioned flaps and laterally sliding flaps are mostly used without adding SCTG and are suitable for high vestibules with thick and wide adjacent keratinized tissue that can be transpositioned. Because of limitations of flap mobility and the numerous alternatives that are now available, these techniques remain in use for single teeth or implants in specific circumstances (**Fig. 12**).

PINHOLE SURGICAL TECHNIQUE

In recent years a novel surgical approach to root coverage, called the pinhole surgical technique, has been gaining exposure. Chao[60] introduced it for Miller class I, II, and III recession defects and reported favorable predictability for root coverage and defect reduction up to 18 months following the procedure.

ROOT SURFACE AND IMPLANT SURFACE TREATMENT

Root or implant surface should be smooth and de-contaminated before receiving the tissue graft. Grooves or notches on the root surfaces should be properly contoured because they create dead spaces between the graft and root surface. Defects, calculus, and restorative materials should be eliminated or reshaped with fine diamond burrs or hand instruments. Root surface should be

thoroughly root planed and conditioned with either citric acid,[61] tetracycline, or ethylenediaminetetra-acetic acid (EDTA). The implant surface can be cleaned with air-power abrasive with sodium bi-carbonate powder and application of tetracycline (**Fig. 13**).

Elimination of endotoxins, demineralization, and removal of the smear layer provide exposure of dentinal tubules, which seems to be essential for new attachment procedures on the root surface.

Citric acid causes a greater degree of morpho-logic alterations than EDTA[62] or tetracycline HCl[63–65] and is considered to be a better root-conditioning agent.

Deviating from the protocol can result in dam-age to the tooth, demineralization, and lack of ce-mentogenesis. Chemical conditioning of the dentin has been shown to stimulate the attach-ment of fibroblasts[65] as well as gingival keratino-cytes, which could favor the reformation of a junctional epithelium.[66]

Some clinical studies have failed to observe improved outcomes of surgical technique when using citric acid.[67]

ALTERNATIVES TO AUTOGENOUS SOFT TISSUE GRAFTS

The concept of avoiding the secondary donor sur-gical site adds great appeal to materials that repre-sent an alternative to autogenous donor sites for soft tissue grafting. Although these new materials

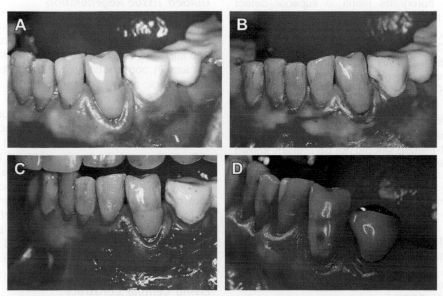

Fig. 12. Lateral sliding flap. (*A*) Canine with an inadequate zone of keratinized tissue. (*B*) Lateral pedicled flap design just before split-thickness dissection. (*C*) Flaps mobilized and sutured into place using 4.0 chromic gut. (*D*) Final result showing an increase in keratinized tissue.

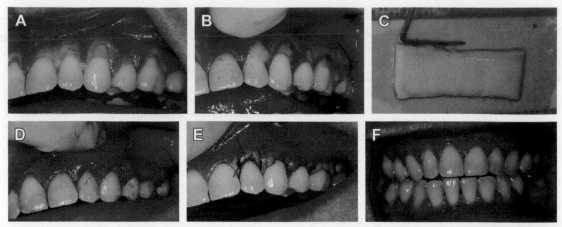

Fig. 13. Allograft for connective tissue graft tunnel. (*A*) Preoperative clinical view showing recession and root exposure. (*B*) Root preparation with EDTA after scaling and root planning. (*C*) Alloderm acellular dermal graft being hydrated and measured. (*D*) Placement of Alloderm into recipient site tunnel preparation without flap elevation. (*E*) Final closure of the coronally advanced flap over the Alloderm. (*F*) Postoperative clinical result, showing complete root coverage in the upper left quadrant.

do not surpass the gold standard (SCTG), they do provide patient satisfaction and esthetics and are available in abundance.

Allograft

Allografts such as acellular dermal matrix (ADM) have been used around teeth and implants to substitute the autogenous connective tissue grafts, especially for larger recipient sites or when obtaining autogenous tissue is not feasible and would lead to much higher postoperative discomfort. Allografts and autografts yield similar predictability for root coverage techniques; however, connective tissue autografts result in superior defect coverage, higher keratinized tissue and attachment gain, and lower residual probing depths (see **Fig. 13**).[68–72]

Allografts also provide an alternative to replace an autogenous free gingival graft (**Fig. 14**).

Wei and colleagues[73,74] conducted a study comparing the effectiveness of ADM and free gingival graft for increasing the width of attached gingiva. The results suggested that tissue formed at the ADM-treated site did not parallel any known mucosa and was more similar to scar tissue.

Xenograft

Xenografts that include thick collagen matrices have been introduced as an alternative to autografts or allografts for use as free gingival or connective tissue grafts.

McGuire and Scheyer[75] showed that xenogeneic collagen matrix with a CAF represents a viable alternative to SCTG in the treatment of recession defects, without the morbidity of soft tissue graft harvest.

In systematic review evaluating esthetic soft tissue management for both teeth and dental implants, xenogeneic collagen matrix was comparable with SCTG in terms of mean keratinized tissue gain; however, it did not achieve the same root coverage.[73]

Similarly, in another systematic review of the most effective techniques for soft tissue management around dental implants, the technique using an animal-derived collagen matrix was able to achieve its goal, but at the cost of a worsened esthetic outcome.[30]

Guided Tissue Regeneration

Guided tissue regeneration (GTR) has been used for treatment of recession defects around teeth and implants using resorbable and nonresorbable barriers in combination with various bone grafts and biologic agents.

GTR-based root coverage can be used successfully to repair gingival recession defects. However, most studies that compared GTR and SCTG concluded that SCTG resulted in statistically better root coverage, width of keratinized gingiva, and complete root coverage.[76–79] Ten-year follow-up comparing SCTG and GTR for root coverage found that the long-term stability of root coverage (ie, the reduction of recession depth) and esthetic results perceived by patients were significantly better using SCTG compared with GTR surgery using bioabsorbable barriers.[80]

Living Cellular Construct

Living cellular constructs (LCC) are derived from autogenous or allogenic sources.

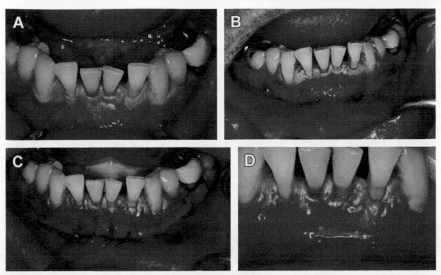

Fig. 14. Allograft for free gingival graft (*A*) Anterior mandibular preoperative view showing a narrow zone of keratinized tissue. (*B*) Subperiosteal dissection in preparation for Alloderm augmentation. Note that the flap has been sutured inferiorly to the apical periosteum. (*C*) Operative view showing the Alloderm secured in place over the periosteal bed with interrupted and sling sutures. (*D*) Eight-week postoperative view showing an increased zone of keratinized tissue.

Platelet-rich fibrin (PRF) is of autologous origin and has been reported in the literature as being used for enhancing healing of the palatal donor site[81] and for papilla reconstruction.[23]

PRF was also used to treat multiple gingival recessions.[82] The natural fibrin architecture of PRF seems responsible for releasing large amounts of growth factors and matrix glycoproteins. These biochemical components of PRF are involved in wound healing and tissue regeneration.[83] The

addition of PRF to a CAF in treatment of Miller class I and II recession defects resulted in superior root coverage compared with CAF alone.[84]

Search of site-appropriate tissue in the oral cavity has included application of living cellular sheet (LCS) in oral soft tissue therapy as a free gingival graft.[85,86]

LCS is an allogenic graft composed of cultured keratinocytes and fibroblasts in bovine collagen and has been used for more than 14 years to treat patients with cutaneous wounds.[87–90] (**Fig. 15**).

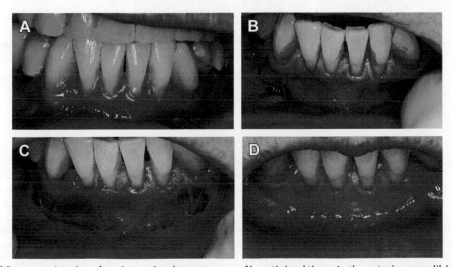

Fig. 15. (*A*) Preoperative view showing an inadequate zone of keratinized tissue in the anterior mandible. (*B*) Supraperiosteal dissection completed in order to receive the graft. Note that the flap is secured inferiorly to the apical periosteum. (*C*) The Mucograft is sutured into place using a combination of interrupted and sling sutures in order to ensure graft immobility. (*D*) Final 12-week postoperative result showing an increased zone of keratinized tissue.

Based on histologic findings, the authors suggested that LCS-treated sites resembled gingiva rather than alveolar mucosa. Compared with sites treated with autogenous grafts, tissue generated at LCS-treated sites presented with more site-appropriate tissue that was deemed superior in terms of color and texture match to adjacent untreated tissue, absence of scar formation, or keloidlike appearance as well as mucogingival junction alignment. Besides superior esthetics, LCC also scored better in patient satisfaction; however it was inferior to free gingival graft in comparisons of the mean keratinized tissue gain.[69]

Biologic agents

Biologic agents have been explored in conjunction with soft tissue grafting to improve migration and differentiation of cells in grafted sites. The data from systematic review by Fu and colleagues[69] concluded that the adjunctive use of biologic agents did not exert a significant effect on mean root coverage and mean amount of keratinized tissue gain.

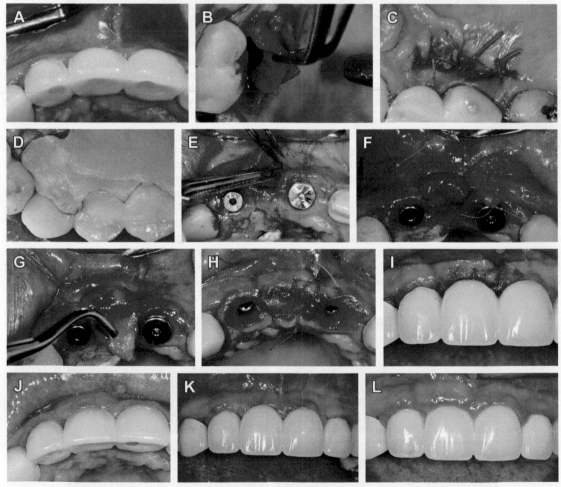

Fig. 16. SCTG ridge augmentation. (*A*) Preoperative view showing an inadequate bucolingual dimension under pontic #8 in the anterior maxilla. (*B*) Intraoperative view showing harvesting of SCTG from the palatal donor site by single-incision approach. (*C, D*) Donor site sutured (*C*) and covered with periodontal dressing (*D*). (*E*) Split-thickness dissection for recipient site preparation using single vertical incision and tunnel preparation. Care was taken to avoid disruption of gingival collars surrounding implants. (*F, G*) Sutures (*arrows*) were used to facilitate advancement of the graft into the recipient site. (*H, I*) SCTG sutured to recipient site before (*H*) and after (*I*) the reinsertion of the implant-supported temporary prosthesis. (*J*) Healing after 8 weeks. Placement of connective tissue graft augmented soft tissue support on the facial aspect of pontic #8. (*K, L*) Placement of connective tissue graft in edentulous area enhanced the esthetics, volume of soft tissue, and papillae under the implant-supported provisional prosthesis as shown by comparing before (*K*) and 8 weeks following surgery (*L*).

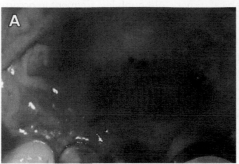
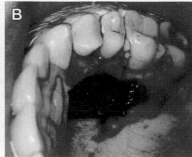

Fig. 17. (*A*) Surgicel is sutured to the donor site. (*B*) Application of a hemostatic agent made of an oxidized polyanhydroglucuronic acid is easy and effective in improving hemostasis.

SOFT TISSUE GRAFTS FOR RIDGE AUGMENTATION

Soft tissue grafts can be used for ridge augmentation to improve esthetics and enhance pontic adaptation (See **Fig. 16**).

Seibert[91,92] presented a classification of ridge deformities and described a full-thickness onlay grafting technique. Other investigators described the use of connective tissue grafts to restore defects in buccolingual dimension.[93–96] Allen and colleagues[97] established that, following surgery, shrinkage was complete in 6 weeks and SCTG remains volumetrically stable over several years.

Miller[98] described a surgical technique using 1 vertical incision creating a tunnel between soft tissue and bone, and inserting into it a connective tissue graft to augment deficient alveolar ridge. This technique is useful for management of soft or hard tissue defects under existing restorations on teeth or implants as well as improving soft tissue support around new ones.

Donor and Recipient Wound Site Protection

Donor sites often present with more postoperative complications than recipient sites. Techniques for protection of donor sites include removable

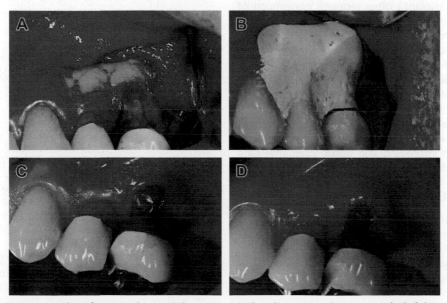

Fig. 18. (*A*) Free gingival graft sutured to recipient site. (*B*) The placement of dressing is helpful in maintaining vestibular depth and protecting the recipient site. (*C*) No root coverage is attempted for Miller class IV soft tissue defect. (*D*) Placement of free gingival graft augmented the amount of keratinized gingiva and improved vestibular depth, as is evident when comparing before (*C*) and 4 weeks following surgery (*D*).

devices or application of materials that stabilize the clot and facilitate wound healing.

Removable devices for the palate include stents made from polymethyl methacrylate or vacuum-formed thermoplastic material as well as existing orthodontic retainers or dentures. Properly fabricated palatal stents should be secure and tightly adhering to palatal tissue. The stent is important for larger and thicker grafts and it dramatically reduces postoperative bleeding and discomfort. Patients with a tendency for slower healing, including smokers,[99] make good candidates for the use of stents (**Fig. 17**).

Materials used most frequently on palatal donor sites include oxidized cellulose (Surgicel) and PRF.[81,100] They have been credited as aiding in healing and also adding to procedure time and cost. Periodontal dressing can be applied over smaller donor sites for SCTGs (**Fig. 18**).

Recipient sites can also be covered by a protective barrier. Cyanoacrylate tissue adhesive is applied in a thin layer over the junction of recipient site and graft once the graft is sutured in place. Reports using cyanoacrylate in the oral environment have shown favorable healing and improved hemostasis[101–103] and it has a safe record for intraoral use.[104] Periodontal dressing offers good adaptation over grafted areas and can be helpful in maintaining an increased vestibular depth obtained with surgery.

SUMMARY

Esthetic appearance and functional longevity for teeth and implants often requires conversion of unfavorable soft tissue traits to more favorable ones. Improvement of tissue quality and quantity can be accomplished with many different techniques and materials and largely depends on clinical presentation of the case and familiarity of the clinician with the procedures and materials available. Identification of causal factors, selection of appropriate surgical technique, and evidence-based material selection lead to predictable success when improving soft tissue characteristics around teeth or implants.

ACKNOWLEDGMENTS

The authors thank the following graduate students at Virginia Commonwealth University for their contributions of photographs for this publication: Dr Anya Rost, Dr Fadi Hassan, Dr Sarmad Bakuri, Dr Diego A. Camacho, and Dr Nicholas Kain.

REFERENCES

1. Kennedy JE, Bird WC, Palcanis KG, et al. A longitudinal evaluation of varying widths of attached gingiva. J Clin Periodontol 1985;12(8): 667–75.

2. Wennstrom JL, Lindhe J. Role of attached gingiva for maintenance of periodontal health. Healing following excisional and grafting procedures in dogs. J Clin Periodontol 1983;10(2):206–21.

3. Block MS, Kent JN. Factors associated with soft- and hard-tissue compromise of endosseous implants. J Oral Maxillofac Surg 1990;48(11):1153–60.

4. Wennstrom JL. Lack of association between width of attached gingiva and development of soft tissue recession. A 5-year longitudinal study. J Clin Periodontol 1987;14(3):181–4.

5. Bangazi F, Wennstrom JL, Lekholm U. Recession of the soft tissue margin at oral implants. A 2-year longitudinal prospective study. Clin Oral Implants Res 1996;7(4):303–10.

6. Warren K, Buser D, Lang NP, et al. Plaque-induced peri-implantitis in the presence or absence of keratinized mucosa. Clin Oral Implants Res 1995;6:131.

7. Silness J, Loe H. Periodontal disease in pregnancy. II. Correlation between oral hygiene and periodontal condition. Acta Odontol Scand 1964;22: 121–35.

8. Friedman N. Mucogingival surgery. Tex Dent J 1957;75:358–62.

9. Miller PD Jr. Regenerative and reconstructive periodontal plastic surgery. Dent Clin North Am 1988; 32:287–306.

10. Genco RJ, Newman MG. Consensus report-mucogingival therapy Ann Periodontol 1996;1: 702–6

11. Chu SJ, Tarnow DP. Managing esthetic challenges with anterior implants. Part 1: midfacial recession defects from etiology to resolution. Compend Contin Educ Dent 2013;34(7):26–31.

12. Sullivan HC, Atkins JH. Free autogenous gingival grafts. III. Utilization of grafts III. Utilization of grafts in the treatment of recession. J Periodontol 1968;6:153.

13. Miller PD. A classification of marginal tissue recession. Int J Periodontics Restorative Dent 1985;5:9.

14. Armitage GC. Development of a classification system for periodontal diseases and conditions. Ann Periodontol 1999;4(1):1–6.

15. Kokich VO, Kokich VG, Kiyak HA. Perceptions of dental professionals and laypersons to altered dental esthetics: asymmetric and symmetric situations. Am J Orthod Dentofacial Orthop 2006; 130(2):141–51.

16. Chu SJ, Tan JH, Stappert CF, Tarnow DP. Gingival zenith positions and levels of the maxillary anterior dentition. J Esthet Restor Dent 2009;21(2):113–20.

17. Kan JY, Rungcharassaeng K, Umezu K, et al. Dimensions of peri-implant mucosa: an evaluation of maxillary anterior single implants in humans. J Periodontol 2003;74(4):557–62.

18. Schneider D, Grunder U, Ender A, et al. Volume gain and stability of peri-implant tissue following bone and soft tissue augmentation: 1-year results from a prospective cohort study. Clin Oral Implants Res 2011;22(1):28–37.

19. Esposito M, Ekestubbe A, Gröndahl K. Radiological evaluation of marginal bone loss at tooth surfaces facing single Brånemark implants. Clin Oral Implants Res 1993;4(3):151–7.

20. Tarnow DP, Cho SC, Wallace SS. The effect of inter-implant distance on the height of inter-implant bone crest. J Periodontol 2000;71(4):546–9.

21. Chocquet V, Hermans M, Adriaenssens P, et al. Clinical and radiographic evaluation of the papilla level adjacent to single-tooth implants. A retrospective study in the maxillary anterior region. J Periodontol 2001;72:1364–71.

22. Tarnow DP, Magner AW, Fletcher P. The effect of the distance from the contact point to the crest of bone on the presence or absence of the interproximal dental papilla. J Periodontol 1992; 63(12):995–6.

23. Arunachalam LT, Merugu S, Sudhakar U. A novel surgical procedure for papilla reconstruction using platelet rich fibrin. Contemp Clin Dent 2012;3(4): 467–70.

24. Becker W, Gabitov I, Stepanov M, et al. Minimally invasive treatment for papillae deficiencies in the esthetic zone: a pilot study. Clin Implant Dent Relat Res 2010;12:1–0.

25. Jaiswal P, Bhongade M, Tiwari I, et al. Surgical reconstruction of interdental papilla using subepithelial connective tissue graft (SCTG) with a coronally advanced flap: a clinical evaluation of five cases. J Contemp Dent Pract 2010;11(6):E049–57.

26. Tarnow D, Elian N, Fletcher P, et al. Vertical distance from the crest of bone to the height of the interproximal papilla between adjacent implants. J Periodontol 2003;74(12):1785–8.

27. Schropp L, Isidor F. Papilla dimension and soft tissue level after early vs. delayed placement of single-tooth implants: 10-year results from a randomized controlled clinical trial. Clin Oral Implants Res 2015;26(3):278–86.

28. Gallucci GO, Mavropoulos A, Bernard JP, et al. Influence of immediate implant loading on peri-implant soft tissue morphology in the edentulous maxilla. Int J Oral Maxillofac Implants 2007;22(4): 595–602.

29. Kois JC, Kan JY. Predictable peri-implant gingival aesthetics: surgical and prosthodontic rationales. Pract Proced Aesthet Dent 2001;13(9):691–8.

30. Esposito M, Maghaireh H, Grusovin MG, et al. Soft tissue management for dental implants: what are the most effective techniques? A Cochrane systematic review. Eur J Oral Implantol 2012;5(3): 221–38.

31. Yoshino S, Kan JY, Rungcharassaeng K, et al. Effects of connective tissue grafting on the facial gingival level following single immediate implant placement and provisionalization in the esthetic zone: a 1-year randomized controlled prospective study. Int J Oral Maxillofac Implants 2014;29(2): 432–40.

32. Grunder U. Crestal ridge width changes when placing implants at the time of tooth extraction with and without soft tissue augmentation after a healing period of 6 months: report of 24 consecutive cases. Int J Periodontics Restorative Dent 2011;31(1):9–17.

33. Deeb GR, Deeb JG, Agarwal V, et al. Use of transalveolar sutures to maintain vestibular depth and manipulate keratinized tissue following alveolar ridge reduction and implant placement for mandibular prosthesis. J Oral Maxillofac Surg 2015;73(1): 48–52.

34. Dorfman HS, Kennedy JE, Bird WC. Longitudinal evaluation of free autogenous gingival grafts. A four year report. J Periodontol 1982;53(6):349–52.

35. Jahnke PV, Sandifer JB, Gher ME, et al. Thick free gingival and connective tissue autografts for root coverage. J Periodontol 1993;64(4):315–22.

36. Nabers JM. Free gingival grafts. Periodontics 1966; 4:243.

37. Pennel B, Tabor J, King K, et al. Free masticatory mucosa graft. J Periodontol 1969;40:162–6.

38. Sullivan H, Atkins J. Free autogenous gingival grafts. III. Utilization of grafts in the treatment of gingival recession. Periodontics 1968;6:152–60.

39. Rateitschak KH, Egli U, Fringeli G. Recession: a 4-year longitudinal study after free gingival grafts. J Clin Periodontol 1979;6(3):158–64.

40. Miller PD. Root coverage using the free soft tissue autograft following citric acid application. III. A successful and predictable procedure in areas of deep-wide recession. Int J Periodontics Restorative Dent 1985;5(2):14–37.

41. Matter J, Cimasoni G. Creeping attachment after free gingival grafts. J Periodontol 1976;47(10): 574–9.

42. Langer B, Calagna L. The alteration of lingual mucosa with free gingival grafts. Protection of a denture bearing surface. J Periodontol 1978;49(12): 646–8.

43. Holbrook T, Ochsenbein C. Complete coverage of denuded root surface with a one stage gingival graft. Int J Periodontics Restorative Dent 1983;3:8.

44. Bernimoulin J. Coronally repositioned periodontal flap. Clinical evaluation after one year. J Clin Periodontol 1975;2:1.

45. Karring T, Ostergaard E, Löe H. Conservation of tissue specificity after heterotopic transplantation of gingiva and alveolar mucosa. J Periodontal Res 1971;6:282–93.

46. Karring T, Lang NP, Löe H. The role of gingival connective tissue in determining epithelial differentiation. J Periodontal Res 1975;10:1–11.

47. Burkhardt R, Joss A, Lang NP. Soft tissue dehiscence coverage around endosseous implants: a prospective cohort study. Clin Oral Implants Res 2008;19(5):451–7.

48. Zucchelli G, Mazzotti C, Mounssif I, et al. A novel surgical-prosthetic approach for soft tissue dehiscence coverage around single implant. Clin Oral Implants Res 2013;24(9):957–62.

49. Hsu YT, Shieh CH, Wang HL. Using soft tissue graft to prevent mid-facial mucosal recession following immediate implant placement. J Int Acad Periodontol 2012;14(3):76–82.

50. Langer B, Calagna L. The subepithelial connective tissue graft. J Prosthet Dent 1980;44(4):363–7.

51. Mörmann W, Schaer F, Firestone AR. The relationship between success of free gingival grafts and transplant thickness. Revascularization and shrinkage–a one year clinical study. J Periodontol 1981;52(2):74–80.

52. Reiser GM, Bruno JF, Mahan PE, et al. The subepithelial connective tissue graft palatal donor site: anatomic considerations for surgeons. Int J Periodontics Restorative Dent 1996;16(2):130–7.

53. Raetzke PB. Covering localized areas of root exposure employing the "envelope" technique. J Periodontol 1985;56(7):397–402.

54. Harris RJ, Miller LH, Harris CR, et al. A comparison of three techniques to obtain root coverage on mandibular incisors. J Periodontol 2005;76(10): 1758–67.

55. Langer B, Langer L. Subepithelial connective tissue graft technique for root coverage. J Periodontol 1985;56(12):715–20.

56. Cordioli G, Mortarino C, Chierico A, et al. Comparison of 2 techniques of subepithelial connective tissue graft in the treatment of gingival recessions. J Periodontol 2001;72(11):1470–6.

57. Bouchard P, Etienne D, Ouhayoun JP, et al. Subepithelial connective tissue grafts in the treatment of gingival recessions. A comparative study of 2 procedures. J Periodontol 1994;65(10):929–36.

58. Harris RJ. Histologic evaluation of connective tissue grafts in humans. Int J Periodontics Restorative Dent 2003;23(6):575–83.

59. Harris RJ. Connective tissue grafts combined with either double pedicle grafts or coronally positioned pedicle grafts: results of 266 consecutively treated defects in 200 patients. Int J Periodontics Restorative Dent 2002;22(5):463–71.

60. Chao JC. A novel approach to root coverage: the pinhole surgical technique. Int J Periodontics Restorative Dent 2012;32(5):521–31.

61. Miller PD Jr. Root coverage using a free soft tissue autograft following citric acid application. Part 1: technique. Int J Periodontics Restorative Dent 1982;2(1):65–70.

62. Prasad SS, Radharani C, Varma S, et al. Effects of citric acid and EDTA on periodontally involved root surfaces: a SEM study. J Contemp Dent Pract 2012;13(4):446–51.

63. Balos K, Bal B, Eren K. The effects of various agents on root surfaces (a scanning electron microscopy study). Newsl Int Acad Periodontol 1991;1(2):13–6.

64. Labahn R, Fahrenbach WH, Clark SM, et al. Root dentin morphology after different modes of citric acid and tetracycline hydrochloride conditioning. J Periodontol 1992;63(4):303–9.

65. Babay N. Attachment of human gingival fibroblasts to periodontally involved root surface following scaling and/or etching procedures: a scanning electron microscopy study. Braz Dent J 2001; 12(1):17–21.

66. Vanheusden AJ, Goffinet G, Zahedi S, et al. In vitro stimulation of human gingival epithelial cell attachment to dentin by surface conditioning. J Periodontol 1999;70(6):594–603.

67. Caffesse RG, De LaRosa M, Garza M, et al. Citric acid demineralization and subepithelial connective tissue grafts. J Periodontol 2000;71(4):568–72.

68. Hirsch A, Goldstein M, Goultschin J, et al. 2-year follow-up of root coverage using sub-pedicle acellular dermal matrix allografts and subepithelial connective tissue autografts. J Periodontol 2005;76(8): 1323–8.

69. Fu JH, Su CY, Wang HL. Esthetic soft tissue management for teeth and implants. J Evid Based Dent Pract 2012;12(3 Suppl):129–42.

70. Harris RJ. A short-term and long-term comparison of root coverage with an acellular dermal matrix and a subepithelial graft. J Periodontol 2004;75: 734–43.

71. Harris RJ. Acellular dermal matrix used for root coverage: 18 month follow-up observation. Int J Periodontics Restorative Dent 2002;22:156–63.

72. Paolantonio M, Dolci M, Esposito P, et al. Subpedicle acellular dermal matrix graft and autogenous connective tissue graft in the treatment of gingival recessions: a comparative 1-year clinical study. J Periodontol 2002;73:1299–307.

73. Wei PC, Laurell L, Geivelis M, et al. Acellular dermal matrix allografts to achieve increased attached gingiva. Part 1. A clinical study. J Periodontol 2000;71:1297–305.

74. Wei PC, Laurell L, Lingen MW, et al. Acellular dermal matrix allografts to achieve increased attached gingiva. Part 2. A histological comparative study. J Periodontol 2002;73:257–65.

75. McGuire MK, Scheyer ET. Xenogeneic collagen matrix with coronally advanced flap compared to connective tissue with coronally advanced flap for

the treatment of dehiscence-type recession defects. J Periodontol 2010;81:1108–17.

76. Al-Hamdan K, Eber R, Sarment D, et al. Guided tissue regeneration-based root coverage: meta-analysis. J Periodontol 2003;74(10):1520–33.

77. Oates TW, Robinson M, Gunsolley JC. Surgical therapies for the treatment of gingival recession. A systematic review. Ann Periodontol 2003;8(1):303–20.

78. Tatakis DN, Trombelli L. Gingival recession treatment: guided tissue regeneration with bio-absorbable membrane versus connective tissue graft. J Periodontol 2000;71(2):299–307.

79. Jepsen K, Heinz B, Halben JH, et al. Treatment of gingival recession with titanium reinforced barrier membranes versus connective tissue grafts. J Periodontol 1998;69(3):383–91.

80. Nickles K, Ratka-Krüger P, Neukranz E, et al. Ten-year results after connective tissue grafts and guided tissue regeneration for root coverage. J Periodontol 2010;81(6):827–36.

81. Jain V, Triveni MG, Kumar AB, et al. Role of platelet-rich-fibrin in enhancing palatal wound healing after free graft. Contemp Clin Dent 2012;3(Suppl 2):S240–3.

82. Aroca S, Keglevich T, Barbieri B, et al. Clinical evaluation of a modified coronally advanced flap alone or in combination with a platelet rich fibrin membrane for the treatment of adjacent multiple gingival recessions: a 6-month study. J Periodontol 2009;80:244–52.

83. Dohan Ehrenfest DM, Diss A, Odin G, et al. In vitro effects of Choukroun's PRF (platelet-rich fibrin) on human gingival fibroblasts, dermal prekeratinocytes, preadipocytes, and maxillofacial osteoblasts in primary cultures. Oral Surg Oral Med Oral Pathol Oral Radiol Endod 2009;108:341–52.

84. Padma R, Shilpa A, Kumar PA, et al. A split mouth randomized controlled study to evaluate the adjunctive effect of platelet-rich fibrin to coronally advanced flap in Miller's class-I and II recession defects. J Indian Soc Periodontol 2013;17(5):631–6.

85. McGuire MK, Scheyer ET, Nevins ML, et al. Living cellular construct for increasing the width of keratinized gingiva: results from a randomized, within-patient, controlled trial. J Periodontol 2011;82:1414–23.

86. Scheyer ET, Nevins ML, Neiva R, et al. Generation of site-appropriate tissue by a living cellular sheet in the treatment of mucogingival defects. J Periodontol 2014;85(4):57–64.

87. Veves A, Falanga V, Armstrong DG, et al, Apligraf Diabetic Foot Ulcer Study. Graftskin, a human skin equivalent, is effective in the management of noninfected neuropathic diabetic foot ulcers: A prospective randomized multicenter clinical trial. Diabetes Care 2001;24:290–5.

88. Muhart M, McFalls S, Kirsner RS, et al. Behavior of tissue-engineered skin: a comparison of a living skin equivalent, autograft, and occlusive dressing in human donor sites. Arch Dermatol 1999;135:913–8.

89. Waymack P, Duff RG, Sabolinski M, The Apligraf Burn Study Group. The effect of a tissue engineered bilayered living skin analog, over meshed split-thickness autografts on the healing of excised burn wounds. Burns 2000;26:609–19.

90. Falanga V, Margolis D, Alvarez O, et al, Human Skin Equivalent Investigators Group. Rapid healing of venous ulcers and lack of clinical rejection with an allogeneic cultured human skin equivalent. Arch Dermatol 1998;134:293–300.

91. Seibert JS. Reconstruction of deformed partially edentulous ridges, using full thickness onlay grafts. Part I. Technique and wound healing. Compend Contin Educ Dent 1983;4:437.

92. Seibert JS. Reconstruction of deformed, partially edentulous ridges, using full thickness onlay grafts. Part II. Prosthetic/periodontal interrelationships. Compend Contin Educ Dent 1983;4:549.

93. Meltzer J. Edentulous area tissue graft correction of an esthetic defect: a case report. J Periodontol 1979;50:320.

94. Langer B, Calagna L. Sub-epithelial graft to correct ridge concavities. J Prosthet Dent 1980;44:363.

95. Garber D, Rosenberg ES. The edentulous ridge in fixed prosthodontics. Compend Contin Educ Dent 1982;1:23.

96. Abrams L. Augmentation of the deformed residual edentulous ridge for fixed prosthesis. Compend Contin Educ Dent 1980;1:205.

97. Allen EP, Gainza CS, Farthing GG, et al. Improved technique for localized ridge augmentation. J Periodontol 1985;56:195.

98. Miller PD. Ridge augmentation under existing fixed prosthesis: simplified technique. J Periodontol 1986;57(12):742–5.

99. Silva CO, Ribeiro Edel P, Sallum AW, et al. Free gingival grafts: graft shrinkage and donor-site healing in smokers and non-smokers. J Periodontol 2010;81(5):692–701.

100. Kulkarni MR, Thomas BS, Varghese JM, et al. Platelet-rich fibrin as an adjunct to palatal wound healing after harvesting a free gingival graft: a case series. J Indian Soc Periodontol 2014;18(3):399–402.

101. Habib A, Mehanna A, Medra A. Cyanoacrylate: a handy tissue glue in maxillofacial surgery: our experience in Alexandria, Egypt. J Maxillofac Oral Surg 2013;12(3):243–7.

102. Joshi AD, Saluja H, Mahindra U, et al. A comparative study: efficacy of tissue glue and sutures after impacted mandibular third molar removal. J Maxillofac Oral Surg 2011;10(4):310–5.

103. Idle MR, Monaghan AM, Lamin SM, et al. N-butyl-2-cyanoacrylate (NBCA) tissue adhesive as a haemostatic agent in a venous malformation of the mandible. Br J Oral Maxillofac Surg 2013;51(6): 565–7.

104. Inal S, Yilmaz N, Nisbet C, et al. Biochemical and histopathological findings of N-butyl-2-cyanoacrylate in oral surgery: an experimental study. Oral Surg Oral Med Oral Pathol Oral Radiol Endod 2006;102(6):14–7.

Surgical Treatment of Impacted Canines
What the Orthodontist Would Like the Surgeon to Know

Adrian Becker, BDS, LDS, DDO*, Stella Chaushu, DMD, MSc, PhD

KEYWORDS

- Impacted canine • Surgical exposure • Open or closed exposure • Attachment bonding
- Immediate traction • Steel ligature connector

KEY POINTS

- If there is an existing malocclusion that requires orthodontic treatment, a full orthodontic appraisal is needed for planning the overall mechanotherapy.
- It is incumbent on the oral and maxillofacial surgeon and the orthodontist to evaluate the 3-dimensional location of the tooth and assess whether the tooth or teeth are salvageable.
- Excepting the very simplest and mildest forms of impaction, orthodontics will be necessary to properly resolve the impaction and align the tooth.

 Videos of two very high impacted canines using cone beam computed tomography accompany this article at http://www.oralmaxsurgery.theclinics.com/. One is located high on the palatal side of the incisor root apices and the second in the line of the arch, high above the premolar with interference from abnormal premolar roots

INTRODUCTION

When an impacted permanent maxillary canine has been diagnosed, the general practitioner or pediatric dentist typically thinks in terms of surgery and orthodontics and, usually, in that order. Thus, the patient is frequently referred to the oral surgeon in the first instance.

In this scenario, a "surgery first" approach can achieve several important goals.

1. By exposing the tooth to the oral environment, surgery can provide a way for autonomous natural eruption.
2. Surgery could simplify orthodontic treatment that would then be delayed for several months if, as advocated by the late Vince Kokich, exposure and packing of the exposure wound would

encourage autonomous eruption of the canine.[1,2]
3. A supernumerary tooth or odontome that has impeded the normal eruption of the tooth could be removed.
4. Access to the tooth may be provided for the later placement of an attachment and for the application of traction if rehealing of the tissues over the crown is prevented using a surgical/periodontal pack over the open wound or by apically repositioning a surgical flap higher up on the crown of the exposed tooth.

However, surgery alone is limited when:

1. Space is inadequate in the dental arch to accommodate the impacted tooth, thereby impeding its natural eruption.

Department of Orthodontics, Hebrew University-Hadassah School of Dental Medicine, 6 Shalom Aleichem Street, Apartment #3, Jerusalem 92148, Israel
* Corresponding author.
E-mail address: adrian.becker@mail.huji.ac.il

Oral Maxillofacial Surg Clin N Am 27 (2015) 449–458
http://dx.doi.org/10.1016/j.coms.2015.04.007
1042-3699/15/$ – see front matter © 2015 Elsevier Inc. All rights reserved.

2. To maintain a patent exposure, an excessive amount of gingival tissue and bone must be removed, to the detriment of the periodontal outcome.[3–5]

3. Autonomous eruption is unlikely to occur and the surgeon feels the necessity for a much more radical open exposure and/or the tooth is "gently" elevated to "free" it from the surrounding tissues, or if bone channeling is performed. These procedures are highly suspect for inflicting irreversible damage to the periodontium[4] or the cementum layer of the root.[6]

4. Immediate application of traction cannot be employed because there is no orthodontic appliance or temporary orthodontic bone anchor present, from which to apply the traction force.

5. The tooth needs to be moved away from the root of an adjacent tooth, particularly when there are signs of resorption of that root.[7]

6. The tooth is located in a grossly ectopic site.[8]

Surgery without orthodontic coordination may occasionally result in:

1. The surgeon exposing an impacted tooth before an orthodontic appraisal has been made. This may be one of the teeth that the orthodontist would wish to sacrifice in the course of subsequent orthodontic treatment, because overall and comprehensive considerations may demand the remedial extraction of 4 permanent teeth.

2. Rehealing of the surrounding tissues over the exposed tooth, making it once again inaccessible.

3. The surgeon bonding an attachment to an aspect of the crown of the tooth in a strategically incorrect position during the operation, which may make subsequent orthodontic traction difficult to direct or control.

4. Poor timing, because active traction may be impossible to apply for several months or years, during which reburial of the tooth may still occur.

5. A successful treatment from the surgical and orthodontic standpoints, but that may become a periodontal disaster if the root apex of an impacted tooth is in a severely displaced initial location. The orthodontist may consider that, although it may be possible to achieve a good orthodontic resolution of the impaction and alignment of the tooth into its place in the dental arch, the periodontal prognosis may be compromised, after the difficult orthodontic root movements of the tooth, with the outcome showing insufficient bony support, poor soft tissue cover, and an unsightly and elongated clinical crown.

6. Committing the patient to orthodontic treatment, because this is the "best" line of treatment, but for which he or she may not be prepared. Perhaps oral hygiene is poor or there is frank caries in other teeth, or simply that the patient is unwilling or financially unprepared to wear braces.

THE ORTHODONTIST MUST BE THE "MASTER OF CEREMONIES"

If there is an existing malocclusion that requires orthodontic treatment, a full orthodontic appraisal is needed for planning the overall mechanotherapy. The orthodontist will undertake a clinical examination, including plaster casts and the routine radiographs needed for any orthodontic case. For a patient with an impacted maxillary canine, there will be the additional requirement of accurately locating the impacted tooth in 3 planes of space and in relation to the adjacent teeth. Further radiography, together with cone beam CT, will often be required to diagnose resorption of the roots of the incisors and to confirm the integrity of the outline and texture of the impacted tooth itself.[9,10]

When all the information is collated, a treatment plan will be formulated to resolve the overall malocclusion and to decide the future of the impacted tooth, which may lead to a decision to extract permanent teeth. In general, the choice of tooth for extraction devolves on a premolar in each quadrant. However, no tooth is sacrosanct and, if the choice is between an erupted healthy premolar and a deeply buried canine in an ectopic location, whose periodontal outcome may be compromised in the final analysis, the canine should be extracted.[4]

Excepting the very simplest and mildest forms of impaction, orthodontics will be necessary to resolve properly the impaction and align the tooth. This being so, the dental arches need to be aligned and leveled and adequate space provided in the canine location, to place a heavy archwire in the bracket slots and, thus, to establish a sound anchorage base from which to apply traction to the tooth. This preparatory step takes time—occasionally, as much as a year or more—but orthodontists are well-practiced at achieving these goals.

Clearly then, the orthodontist is the person who is ultimately responsible to the patient for the success of the treatment plan as a whole. The oral and maxillofacial surgeon is responsible only for the success of the immediate operative procedure, in which he or she provides access to the tooth, previously denied. It is incumbent on both the oral and maxillofacial surgeon and the orthodontist to evaluate the 3-dimensional location of the tooth and, together, assess whether the tooth or teeth are salvageable. If the canine position is beyond reasonable bounds, extraction will be advised. For the oral and maxillofacial surgeon, an assessment of the location of the crown of the canine in the 3 planes of space and in relation to the roots of the adjacent teeth is essential, because the surgeon is only interested in exposing the crown and preventing damage to the adjacent teeth. Orientation of the root of the tooth is not relevant to his or her ability to achieve success in the exposure procedure.

For the orthodontist, the assessment also involves the 3-dimensional orientation of the long axis of the tooth and an exact positional diagnosis of its root apex. If the apex is in the line of the arch in the buccolingual plane and in the mesiodistal plane, then the crown of the tooth will only need to be tipped into its place in the arch, a relatively simple biomechanical exercise. For as long as the tooth is not fully engaged in the main archwire, no root movements are possible and, thus, any deviation of the location of the apex, particularly in the buccolingual plane, will demand complicated uprighting and torqueing mechanotherapy, which is technically difficult to perform and reduces the periodontal prognosis of the tooth in the long term.[4]

Accordingly, the orthodontist's evaluation as to whether surgical exposure should be undertaken at all must be considered of primary importance. It follows that the surgeon's essential role is to provide optimal conditions for the orthodontist to be able to proceed to apply forces to the tooth in the direction he or she will have planned, to reduce the impaction and align the tooth.

THE SURGICAL PROCEDURE

There are several appropriate surgical procedures that need to be contemplated and these are classified into open procedures and closed procedures. Each method must additionally take into account the elimination of a supernumerary tooth or odontome, if appropriate.

The Palatal Canine and the Open Exposure Technique

The palatal area is composed of tightly bound attached mucosa, which means that a palatally impacted canine that is erupted through it, after an open exposure procedure, will be invested with attached epithelium in the final instance. After this procedure, the canine must be left exposed to the oral environment and care taken to ensure that healing of the adjacent soft tissues will not recover the tooth and again make it inaccessible. This may be done by clearing a broad area of soft tissue, including the entire dental follicle, oral mucosa and bone, down to the cementoenamel junction (CEJ) and placing a surgical pack to cover the area (**Fig. 1**). This pack would normally be left for 2 to 3 weeks in the hope that the tooth remains visible when the pack is removed, and to provide access for later bonding of an attachment in the

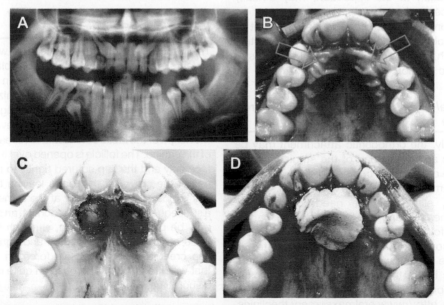

Fig. 1. (*A*) Panoramic view showing palatally impacted maxillary canine and other dental anomalies. (*B*) Occlusal view to show the palpable bulges indicative of relatively superficial, palatally displaced, canines (*arrows*). (*C*) Open exposure of the 2 canines. (*D*) A suture-stabilized periodontal pack covers the exposed area, with the aim of preventing healing over of the palatal soft tissue and maintaining access to the tooth. (Treatment by graduate student Dr O. Yitschaky.)

relative comfort of the orthodontist's office. A word of caution arising from overzealous surgical exposure is at this juncture. To ensure that the tooth does not become recovered by the tissues during the healing period, bone and mucosal tissue are often pared back liberally around the tooth. Together with a complete elimination of the dental follicle, the entire crown down to the CEJ is revealed and a surgical pack placed to maintain the patency of the open exposure site. Exposure of the tooth down to the CEJ and excessive removal of bone and soft tissue will have a detrimental effect on the periodontal outcome of an otherwise successfully treated case, because the junctional epithelium that encircles the cervical few millimeters of crown enamel will be severed irreparably and be pushed apically. The outcome will be seen many months later when the orthodontic treatment has been completed, in the form of a long clinical crown, with loss of bone height, gingival recession, and poor periodontal appearance. On occasion, particularly with the more deeply located teeth, the surgeon will moderately luxate the tooth, with the intention of "loosening it up" or "to check if it is ankylosed" by pushing an elevator beyond the CEJ and into the sensitive cementum covering the root surface. This has been claimed by many to facilitate spontaneous eruption and even to positively redirect its eruption path. However, this common practice, whose intention is to facilitate the orthodontist's later resolution of the impaction, may actually initiate a cervical root resorption process or an ankylotic union at that site. The development of these pathologic entities will then prevent eruption of the tooth, causing the failure of all attempts at orthodontic traction.[6,11]

The Palatal Canine and the Closed Exposure Technique

Alternatively, the orthodontic attachment may be bonded as an integral part of the surgical procedure in the office of the oral and maxillofacial surgeon. This method demands a less radical surgical procedure, eliminating the need for exposure down to the CEJ and leaving the deeper part of the dental follicle intact.[12] This is because contact with and control of the tooth may be maintained through the ligature wire that is tied to the attachment. This is the thinking involved in the closed exposure procedure (**Fig. 2**, Video 1, available online at http://www.oralmaxsurgery.theclinics.com/). In essence, hard and soft tissue preservation, particularly in the CEJ area, and full replacement of the surgical flap create an environment at the completion of treatment, in which the tooth

will still be invested with the same healthy attached gingiva, but the clinical crown length, the gingival level, the alveolar crest height and the periodontal parameters will be much more favorable.[13] This method is particularly useful when the impacted tooth is situated deeply. An open procedure would leave a very wide mucosal deficiency in the palate. Conversely, a superficially palpable canine should be left open after the exposure, with or without a surgical pack as a dressing.

The Labial Canine and the Window Technique

A labially impacted canine, on the other hand, is usually palpable above the level of the attached gingiva and covered only by a thin and mobile oral mucosa. To expose the tooth by opening a semilunar window in the oral mucosa directly over it is very simple, very popular, and often performed by the orthodontist. However, this will result in the tooth being drawn down with no attached gingiva on its labial side and with only this thin, mobile, and easily traumatized covering for its long-term protection (**Fig. 3**). The only time that this is acceptable is when there is a broad band of attached gingiva within which the incision is made, leaving a portion of the thicker tissue above the cut. This will then become the labial gingiva when the tooth is brought into alignment.

There are 2 alternatives to the window technique, each of which will produce superior results in terms of the periodontal health and appearance.

The Labial Canine and the Apically Repositioned Flap Technique

The first is the apically repositioned flap, which is only suitable for the canine which is not displaced mesially or distally from its normal location in the arch. It involves raising a flap from the keratinized gingiva at the crest of the ridge or from the gingival margin of the retained deciduous canine. It is elevated above the height of the labial canine and to reveal the follicle of the canine. The follicle is opened over its labial surface only and the flap sutured tightly to the cervical half of the crown of the tooth, leaving the coronal half exposed (**Fig. 4**). Either at the same time or at a subsequent visit to the orthodontist, an attachment may be placed on the tooth, although the vertical force of the upward-displaced and tightly sutured flap creates a mild extrusive force on the canine that will often improve its position quite markedly in a short time.[14,15]

The Labial Canine and the Closed Exposure Technique

The second alternative is appropriate even in cases where the labial canine is displaced in the

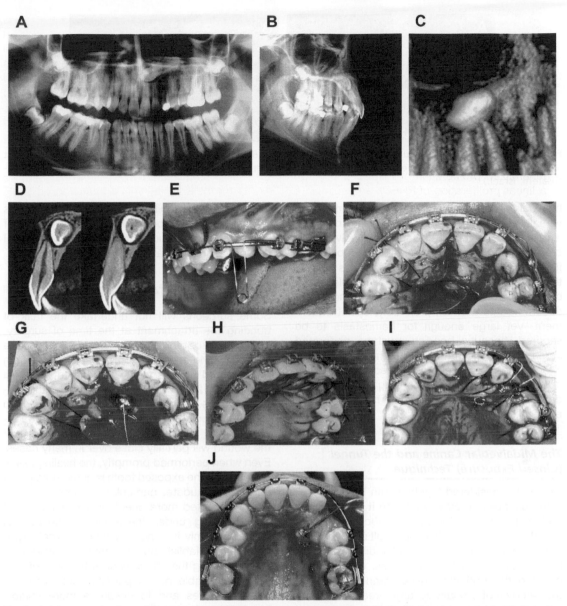

Fig. 2. (A) Panoramic view of impacted maxillary canine high at the level of the incisor root apices. (B) Anterior section of the lateral cephalogram shows the impacted canine in the same long axis as the incisors. (C) A 3-dimensional screen shot extracted from the cone beam CT. (D) Transaxial slices from the cone beam CT to show the relationship of the canine with the central and lateral incisors. (E) The orthodontic setup with the preoperative auxiliary labial archwire in its passive (vertical) state. (F) Minimal exposure of the canine from the palatal aspect. Note that the labial-facing surface of the crown has not been exposed, to avoid exposing the incisor roots. Meticulous hemostasis and moisture control are necessary at this point and are best achieved by the surgeon to enable the orthodontist to perform reliable attachment bonding. (G) With the attachment in place, the ligature exit site must be decided before resuturing. It will be appreciated that the tip of the canine is mesial to the roots of the central incisor and there is no direct route to the canine's location in the arch. (H) The deciduous canine has been extracted and the full flap resutured to its former place. The twisted steel ligature from the bonded attachment pierces the flap overlying the impacted tooth. (I) The active loop of the auxiliary labial archwire is ensnared horizontally in the steel ligature to produce vertical traction. (J) After many months of vertical traction and additional posterior movement of the tooth using a miniscrew in the palate, the tooth has erupted and a new eyelet bonded to its labial surface for its renewed traction in the direction of the main archwire.

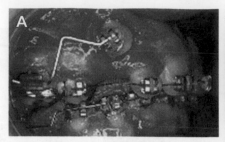
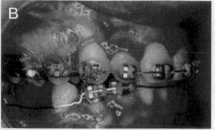

Fig. 3. (*A*) Open surgical exposure through the oral mucosa. (*B*) Successful alignment of the tooth; however, that labial aspect of the tooth is invested with thin and easily ulcerated oral epithelium. (*Courtesy of* Dr G. Engel, Jerusalem, Israel.)

mesiodistal plane, making the technique more universally applicable. The same partial thickness flap is raised from within the keratinized gingiva of the crest of the ridge, as with the apically repositioned flap technique. The follicle of the canine is opened to a very minimal extent over the middle of the crown, with an aperture only large enough to accommodate a small, preferably, eyelet attachment, yet large enough for hemostasis to be secured, because bonding must be performed immediately. The remainder of the follicle is left intact. The attachment is bonded and the gold chain or twisted steel pigtail ligature is drawn downwards and held in place by the sutured edge of the flap.[15,16]

The Midalveolar Canine and the Tunnel (Closed Exposure) Technique

Generally considered together with the labial canines because surgical access to it is performed on the labial side of the alveolar process, the midalveolar impaction is often the result of a mesioangular canine impacting against the distal aspect of the lateral incisor. In these cases, exposing the crown of the tooth in the usual manner will require the removal of a relatively large area of overlying labial plate of bone, which will result in the erupted tooth exhibiting a long, unaesthetic, clinical crown, and reduced bone support on the labial side. Crescini's tunnel technique is an excellent method of

limiting these complications insofar as it erupts the canine down through the evacuated socket of the extracted deciduous canine, leaving the labial part of the socket wall intact (**Fig. 5**).[17]

BONDING THE ATTACHMENT

Some surgeons will not undertake the task of bonding the attachment at the time of surgery, preferring to opt for an open procedure to expose the tooth and then placing a pack to maintain patency and access to the tooth. The pack will be removed 2 to 3 weeks later and the patient returned to the orthodontist to continue orthodontic treatment, including the placement of an attachment on the canine. Inevitably, time elapses and the wound will partially close over in many cases. Even when performed promptly, the healing tissue surrounding the exposed tooth is hemorrhagic and may ooze exudate, particular for those canines that are located more deeply in the palate. Acid etch bonding under these circumstances will almost certainly fail and a second surgical exposure to reestablish access may be necessary. Thus, bonding the attachment at the time of surgery is preferable, both to permit a choice of surgical procedures and to ensure a more reliably bonded attachment.[18]

It goes without saying that a surgeon is perfectly capable to bond an attachment to an exposed tooth! But does the oral and maxillofacial surgeon

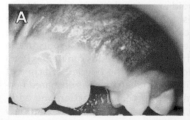
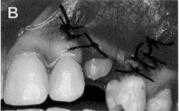
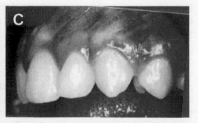

Fig. 4. (*A*) The unerupted canine of this 16-year-old girl has been in this situation for 2 years and has not progressed. (*B*) A flap has been raised from the crest of the ridge incorporating a thick band of attached gingiva and sutured apically on the teeth, exposing half of the crown. (Surgery by Prof L. Shapira.) (*C*) At 9 months postoperatively, the canine has erupted spontaneously, invested with an optimal periodontal environment.

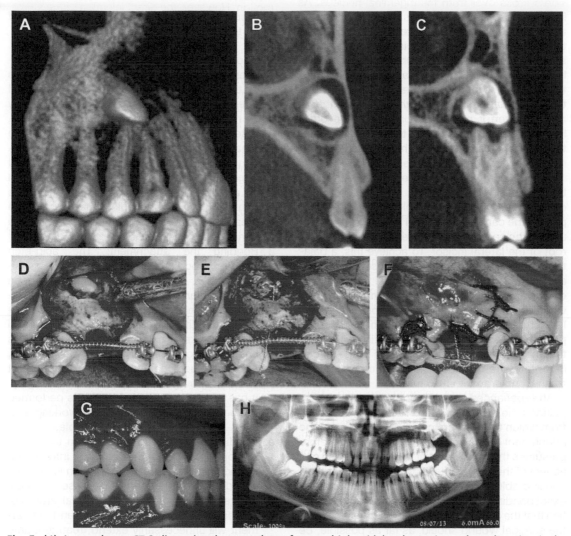

Fig. 5. (*A*) A cone beam CT 3-dimensional screen shot of a very high midalveolar canine, whose location is the result of the mesial curvature on the roots of the first premolar. The deciduous canine has a completely unresorbed root. (*B, C*) Transaxial cone beam CT cuts in the deciduous canine and first premolar areas, respectively, show the relationship between the canine and the premolar roots. (*D*) Orthodontic preparation before surgery was performed to create space in the arch for the canine and the roots of the premolar were moved distally, to distance the apices from the canine eruption path. The illustration shows a full flap raised from the cervical margins of lateral incisor, deciduous canine, and premolar teeth, after extraction of the deciduous canine. The crown of the canine was exposed minimally in the incisal area. (*E*) An eyelet attachment has been bonded to the canine and the twisted stainless steel ligature has been drawn down and through the socket of the extracted deciduous canine, leaving the entire labial wall intact. (*F*) The flap has been sutured back to its former place and traction is applied to the hooked end of the twisted steel ligature by the "swinging gate" offset in the labial archwire. (*G*) The case at completion. (*H*) A panoramic view on the day the orthodontic appliances were removed.

know about the preferred bonding site for the specific case in treatment? Is it important for the attachment to be placed in the midlabial aspect of the canine, just like the brackets on the other teeth, or is it acceptable or even preferable in specific cases to locate it on the palatal, mesial, or distal aspects? Does it matter if it is sited close to the cusp tip or near the cervical area of the crown? How should the gold chain or twisted steel pigtail ligature that is connected to the attachment be made to exit the surgical field? Should this connector be drawn directly toward the space that will have been prepared in the arch or in a different direction? (Video 2, available online at http://www.oralmaxsurgery.theclinics.com/)

Bonding site preference depends entirely on the intended direction of the initial traction force that will be applied to the tooth.[19] For the simpler impactions, where a palatally impacted canine is adjacent to the line of the arch, the tooth needs to be drawn direct to the labial archwire into the space provided. If the attachment in this case is bonded mistakenly to the palatal aspect of the tooth, direct ligation to the archwire will cause the tooth to rotate adversely and end up 180° rotated when it reaches the wire. On the other hand, an attachment sited in the midbuccal position will generate a favorable rotation as the tooth moves toward the archwire.

In direct contrast, should the canine lie mesial to the root of the lateral incisor, which is a frequent occurrence, then this tooth will obstruct the direct path of the canine to the labial archwire. In this situation, the canine must first be distanced from the root of the lateral incisor. To achieve this, a palatally placed attachment will be useful to avoid any rotation, as the tooth is moved in a vertically downward and/or posterior direction.[7] Much later, when the tooth has cleared the obstruction and lies erupted in midpalate with an unobscured path to the archwire, the orthodontist will substitute the attachment for another. This will be placed in a more strategic location on the crown, for the tooth to be drawn to the archwire.

An experienced and skilled orthodontist will have planned the location on the orthodontic appliance from which the traction force will be applied to the attachment on the impacted tooth, which therefore presumes that placement of an attachment on one aspect of the tooth rather than another, will make a considerable difference to the outcome. Both the exact bonding site of the attachment and the direction that the gold chain or twisted steel ligature exits the surgical wound should, as far as possible, be decided in advance to enable the orthodontist to exercise full control over the movement of the tooth. Directional planning of forces is fully in the realm of the orthodontist, who is answerable for both the initial response of the tooth and for its later artistic alignment.

For the orthodontist, the outcome of the surgical episode is of crucial importance and is often the "make or break" factor of the entire treatment plan. Because surgical exposure is a critical procedure where the possibilities for failure are many, it surely behooves the orthodontist to be present even if only in a supervisory capacity.

IT IS ALL A QUESTION OF MAKING THE RIGHT CHOICES

In the light of the many points raised in the foregoing description, we present a list that summarizes the many aspects where choices need to be made to suit the special circumstances surrounding the

orthosurgical modality for the treatment of impacted teeth.

1. Choice of surgical technique: This choice relates to the periodontal outcome and depends on the location of the tooth and on the planned direction of traction, where one technique may be more suited than another.
2. Extent of surgical exposure: Exposure of the area around the CEJ, the unnecessary elimination of the entire dental follicle, when partial removal will suffice, and the aggressive removal of alveolar bone and of the soft tissue is damaging. The more radical the surgery, the greater and the more permanent will be the periodontal consequences.
3. Bonding the attachment: The acid-etch bonding procedure is highly technique sensitive. It is a procedure that an oral surgeon uses quite rarely. To expect the oral and maxillofacial surgeon to bond a small attachment under the conditions of an open, bleeding surgical field and to know exactly where to position it, is unfair and, for the orthodontist, self-defeating. Accidental detachment of a bonded device at the time of surgery will involve repeat surgery. It has been shown that when this is performed by the orthodontist and surgeon working as a team, the procedure is highly reliable.
4. Bonding site selection: Bonding on the wrong site on the crown of the tooth will introduce a rotational component when traction is applied. The degree of rotation will increase markedly before the tooth reaches the labial archwire. Correcting the rotation toward the end of treatment will unnecessarily extend treatment time considerably.
5. Directing the connector: Drawing the gold chain or steel pigtail ligature connector in the wrong direction means either applying traction in the wrong direction or that a second round of surgery will be needed to reorient it.
6. Surgical flap closure: In a closed exposure procedure, the soft tissue flap needs to be sutured back to its former place. In some cases, the connector should be drawn down and held in its place by the sutures at the cut edge of the flap. In others, particularly for a palatal canine that has to avoid the adjacent lateral incisor root, the connector needs to be drawn through the middle of the flap to permit traction in a path that avoids clashing with this potential obstruction.
7. The application of immediate traction: The value of applying traction immediately after the flap is closed, as the last task to be performed in the operating room, should not be underestimated. Immediate force application

using a mechanism that imparts a light force over a wide range can be placed with ease while the patient is anesthetized. In many cases, there is rapid eruption seen at the next visit to the orthodontist. However, the oral and maxillofacial surgeon cannot be expected to place this mechanism and must opt instead for making sure the connector is exposed and not irritant or sharp, leaving activation to the orthodontist at the next visit. This and subsequent adjustments will be much more difficult for the orthodontist to achieve and uncomfortable for the patient to tolerate, and there are many cases for which considerable delay is incurred because of the inability to properly activate a traction mechanism.

This is a very long list of possible bad choices and operational errors of judgment that emanate from ignorance on the part of the surgeon for the requirements of the orthodontist and vice versa, or simply a lack of coordination between the two. Making the wrong choices will lead to longer overall treatment and/or poorer periodontal outcome and even to the difference between success and failure. What can go wrong will go wrong! Thus, any factor that can streamline the treatment must be adopted. None of these prophesies of doom need occur if the orthodontist is present at the surgical procedure as an essential and active member of the team.

IS THIS TREATMENT URGENT?

For the overriding majority of cases, there is no urgency to expose the impacted tooth and time invested in preparing the other teeth to act in concert as a multiple orthodontic anchor base is time well spent. However, the presence of a palatally impacted maxillary canine associated with marked resorption of the root of the adjacent incisor is one of the rare instances that must be considered an orthodontic emergency. In an earlier study, we showed that distancing the canine from the immediate vicinity will effectively arrest the resorption process and will later permit the orthodontic movement of the affected incisor without its undergoing further resorption. Accordingly, in these cases surgery should be arranged as soon as possible, even before the placement of an orthodontic appliance. At the same time the tooth is exposed in the palate and an attachment bonded to the tooth, a miniscrew bone anchor should be placed at a convenient site in the posterior palate. Elastic thread or an elastic chain should then be applied under tension between the steel ligature from the bonded attachment to the head of the miniscrew (**Fig. 6**). This will need to be reapplied 3 or 4 times more until, in favorable circumstances, the palatal tissue bulges as the canine is drawn away from the anterior teeth, to erupt in the midpalatal area.[20] Once the tooth shows positive signs of eruption, a full maxillary fixed orthodontic appliance may be placed. This will need to be reapplied 3 or 4 times more until, in favorable circumstances, the palatal tissue bulges as the canine is drawn away from the anterior teeth, to erupt in the midpalatal area. Once the tooth shows positive signs of movement away from the anterior teeth, a full maxillary fixed orthodontic appliance may be placed, with confidence that further root

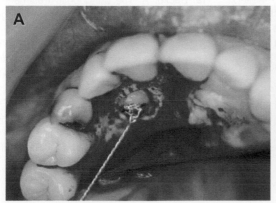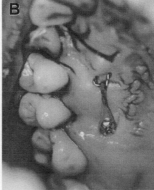

Fig. 6. (*A*) A palatal canine was exposed minimally in an adult patient in whom there was some concern as to whether the tooth would respond to traction. An attachment was bonded to its palatal aspect. (*B*) After fully suturing the flap back to its former place, a miniscrew was inserted in the posterior palate and an elastic chain stretched between the hooked end of the pigtail ligature and the miniscrew, to apply extrusive traction. The elastic chain was changed several times until evidence of canine movement could be seen as a bulge in the palate. Only at that point were orthodontic appliances placed to achieve a successful orthodontic outcome. (*From* Becker A. Orthodontic treatment of impacted teeth. 3rd edition. Oxford (United Kingdom): Wiley Blackwell Publishers; 2012; with permission).

resorption will not occur.[20] This approach may also be used when treating an adult in whom there may be concern that the impacted canine is ankylosed and may not therefore respond to orthodontic traction. With the increased risk of noneruption that exists with advancing age,[21] checking if there will be positive movement of the canine before embarking on expensive orthodontics, may save the patient much time, discomfort, and money.

SUPPLEMENTARY DATA

Supplementary data related to this article can be found online at http://dx.doi.org/10.1016/j.coms.2015.04.007.

REFERENCES

1. Mathews DP, Kokich VG. Palatally impacted canines: the case for preorthodontic uncovering and autonomous eruption. Am J Orthod Dentofacial Orthop 2013;143(4):450–8.

2. Schmidt AD, Kokich VG. Periodontal response to early uncovering, autonomous eruption, and orthodontic alignment of palatally impacted maxillary canines. Am J Orthod Dentofacial Orthop 2007;131(4): 449–55.

3. Becker A, Kohavi D, Zilberman Y. Periodontal status following the alignment of palatally impacted canine teeth. Am J Orthod 1983;84(4):332–6.

4. Kohavi D, Becker A, Zilberman Y. Surgical exposure, orthodontic movement, and final tooth position as factors in periodontal breakdown of treated palatally impacted canines. Am J Orthod 1984;85(1):72–7.

5. Kohavi D, Zilberman Y, Becker A. Periodontal status following the alignment of buccally ectopic maxillary canine teeth. Am J Orthod 1984;85(1):78–82.

6. Becker A, Abramovitz I, Chaushu S. Failure of treatment of impacted canines associated with invasive cervical root resorption. Angle Orthod 2013;83(5): 870–6.

7. Kornhauser S, Abed Y, Harari D, et al. The resolution of palatally impacted canines using palatal-occlusal force from a buccal auxiliary. Am J Orthod Dentofacial Orthop 1996;110(5):528–34.

8. Becker A. Extreme tooth impaction and its resolution. Semin Orthod 2010;16:222–33.

9. Chaushu S, Chaushu G, Becker A. The role of digital volume tomography in the imaging of impacted teeth. World J Orthod 2004;5(2):120–32.

10. Becker A, Chaushu S, Casap-Caspi N. Cone-beam computed tomography and the orthosurgical management of impacted teeth. J Am Dent Assoc 2010;141(Suppl 3):14S–8S.

11. Becker A, Chaushu G, Chaushu S. Analysis of failure in the treatment of impacted maxillary canines. Am J Orthod Dentofacial Orthop 2010;137(6):743–54.

12. Becker A, Chaushu S. Palatally impacted canines: the case for closed surgical exposure and immediate orthodontic traction. Am J Orthod Dentofacial Orthop 2013;143(4):451–9.

13. Chaushu S, Dykstein N, Ben-Bassat Y, et al. Periodontal status of impacted maxillary incisors uncovered by 2 different surgical techniques. J Oral Maxillofac Surg 2009;67(1):120–4.

14. Vanarsdall RL, Corn H. Soft-tissue management of labially positioned unerupted teeth. Am J Orthod 1977;72(1):53–64.

15. Vermette ME, Kokich VG, Kennedy DB. Uncovering labially impacted teeth: apically positioned flap and closed-eruption techniques. Angle Orthod 1995; 65(1):23–32 [discussion: 33].

16. Heaney TG, Atherton JD. Periodontal problems associated with the surgical exposure of unerupted teeth. Br J Orthod 1976;3(2):79–84.

17. Crescini A, Clauser C, Giorgetti R, et al. Tunnel traction of infraosseous impacted maxillary canines. A three-year periodontal follow-up. Am J Orthod Dentofacial Orthop 1994;105(1):61–72.

18. Becker A, Shpack N, Shteyer A. Attachment bonding to impacted teeth at the time of surgical exposure. Eur J Orthod 1996;18(5):457–63.

19. Becker A. The orthodontic treatment of impacted teeth. 3rd edition. Oxford (United Kingdom): Wiley-Blackwell Publishers; 2012.

20. Becker A, Chaushu S. Long-term follow-up of severely resorbed maxillary incisors after resolution of an etiologically associated impacted canine. Am J Orthod Dentofacial Orthop 2005;127(6):650–4 [quiz: 754].

21. Becker A, Chaushu S. Success rate and duration of orthodontic treatment for adult patients with palatally impacted maxillary canines. Am J Orthod Dentofacial Orthop 2003;124(5):509–14.

Preprosthetic Surgery

Hillel Ephros, DMD, MD[a,*], Robert Klein, DDS[b], Anthony Sallustio, DDS[c]

KEYWORDS

• Stability • Retention • Vestibuloplasty • Dental prosthesis • Skin graft • Tuberosity • Torus

KEY POINTS

• The need for preprosthetic surgery may be caused by anatomic variations, gradual loss of supporting tissues, or a lack of foresight during earlier stages of treatment.
• Functional, comfortable, and esthetically pleasing prostheses often require collaboration between the surgeon and restoring dentist.
• All denture bearing hard and soft tissues should be evaluated with great care before denture construction.
• Surgical improvement of existing anatomy should at least be considered in every patient for whom a conventional prosthesis is planned.
• Even the partially implant-borne prosthesis may benefit from preprosthetic surgery.

Preprosthetic surgery comprises a unique and evolving group of soft and hard tissue procedures. Although the focus of such procedures has shifted dramatically over the last 30 years, the fundamental concepts remain unchanged. Preprosthetic surgery exists to serve the needs of dentists who provide patients with replacements for missing teeth and associated tissues. The purpose is to facilitate the fabrication of prostheses or to improve the outcome of prosthodontic treatment. The surgeon's role is to produce an environment in which esthetics and function may be optimized by manipulating, augmenting, or replacing soft and/or hard tissues. With the emergence of implants as predictable anchors for a wide variety of dental prostheses, many preprosthetic procedures, particularly those that were developed to prepare the jaws for dentures, have become less relevant and may be headed toward obsolescence. They have been displaced by a newer set of surgical interventions designed to prepare sites for implant placement. Dr Michael Block reviews these procedures elsewhere in this issue. The discussion that follows provides a historical reference for preprosthetic surgery, focusing on the core concepts and detailing selected procedures that continue to be useful in the successful oral rehabilitation of partially and fully edentulous patients.

GOALS

In the introductory paragraph of his 1972 article "Objectives of Preprosthetic Surgery," Lawson asks: "Why should it be assumed that a full denture is the one type of dental restoration for which the mouth is already perfectly designed?"[1] In fact, the quality of dentures and the patients' experience can often be enhanced significantly by surgical preparation. Oral and maxillofacial surgeons must understand the criteria for successful prostheses and let the needs of patients and the dentist/prosthodontist dictate the selection of applicable preprosthetic procedures. Lawson's criteria include insertion, comfort, retention, stability, adequate occlusion, satisfactory appearance, and no damage to the oral tissues.

The surgical/prosthetic collaboration begins with treatment planning based on diagnostics

---

The authors have nothing to disclose.
[a] Oral and Maxillofacial Surgery, Department of Dentistry, St. Joseph's Regional Medical Center, 703 Main Street, Paterson, NJ 07503, USA; [b] Oral and Maxillofacial Surgery, St. Joseph's Regional Medical Center, 703 Main Street, Paterson, NJ 07503, USA; [c] Prosthodontics and Maxillofacial Prosthetics, St. Joseph's Regional Medical Center, Paterson, NJ 07503, USA
* Corresponding author.
E-mail address: ephrosh@sjhmc.org

Oral Maxillofacial Surg Clin N Am 27 (2015) 459–472
http://dx.doi.org/10.1016/j.coms.2015.04.002
1042-3699/15/$ – see front matter © 2015 Elsevier Inc. All rights reserved.

that are adequate to ensure appropriate procedure selection. These diagnostics should include a thorough clinical examination, mounted study models, and a panoramic radiograph supplemented by periapical films and other imaging as needed. Medical, surgical, anesthetic, and psychological risk assessment should all be done as for any other elective surgery. In the realm of preprosthetic surgery, communication between the surgeon and restoring dentist is crucial. For each of the criteria listed earlier, the team must determine whether existing anatomy is satisfactory and, if not, what intervention might best serve the needs of the patients and the restoring dentist.

- Insertion requires adequate interarch space and a clear path free of bony protuberances, sharp undercuts, and bulbous soft tissue prominences. Applicable procedures may include alveoloplasty, tuberosity reduction, torus, and exostosis removal.
- Comfort is related to the seating of a prosthesis on good-quality soft tissue overlying smooth bone. Examples of procedures that may enhance comfort are alveoloplasty, lingual balcony reduction, removal of redundant soft tissue, frenectomy, and skin graft vestibuloplasty.
- Retention is resistance to vertical displacement and is optimized by an intimate relationship between the prosthesis and the underlying soft tissue. The surface area of contact should be maximized and sealed peripherally. Procedures designed to address retention include frenectomies and various vestibuloplasties.[2]
- Stability is resistance to lateral displacement from functional horizontal and rotational stresses. It depends on adequate ridge height as well as the quantity and quality of soft tissue in the denture-bearing area. In general, severely resorbed maxillae and mandibles are poor candidates for bony augmentation when implants are not part of the restorative plan. When bone is adequate, procedures such as lingual balcony reductions, removal of redundant soft tissue, and skin graft vestibuloplasty may enhance stability.[1,2]
- Adequate occlusion requires a reasonable skeletal relationship between the jaws. For patients with severe skeletal class II or III relationships, orthognathic surgery may be indicated as a preprosthetic procedure.
- Satisfactory appearance is at or near the top of the list of patient expectations and can only be achieved when the restoring dentist is able to set teeth properly in the context of the facial skeleton and overlying soft tissues.

Surgical procedures that address skeletal discrepancies, particularly anteroposterior and vertical issues, may be indicated.

- Damage to the oral tissues must be minimized even with consistent denture use over long periods of time. Maximal denture-bearing surface area distributes the compressive load; high-quality, immobile soft tissue in that area handles that load most effectively. Removal of bony undercuts may allow the masticatory load to be spread as widely as possible. Skin graft vestibuloplasty provides a larger surface area for denture contact and replaces moveable alveolar mucosa with immobile, tough soft tissue that is capable of bearing the masticatory load.

BONY RECONTOURING PROCEDURES
Preoperative Planning

As with any other surgical procedure, planning begins with a thorough history and physical examination. An understanding of patients' surgical and prosthetic expectations must be clear and a determination made as to whether these goals can be achieved.[1] Special emphasis is placed on systemic conditions that may directly affect bone healing. The clinical examination focuses on bony projections and undercuts, large palatal and mandibular tori, and other gross ridge abnormalities. The interarch relationship should be evaluated in 3 dimensions. Radiographs are reviewed for bony pathology, impacted teeth, retained root tips, degree of maxillary sinus pneumatization, and the position of the inferior alveolar canal and mental foramina.[3] This section focuses on bony reduction and recontouring procedures.

Alveoloplasty

Alveolar bone irregularities may be found at the time of tooth extraction or after healing and remodeling has occurred. The goal for alveoloplasty is to achieve optimal tissue support for the planned prosthesis, while preserving as much bone and soft tissue as possible.[4]

1. An incision along the crest of the alveolus, or a sulcular incision before tooth extractions, is created with adequate extension to allow proper visualization of the area of interest. Generally, extension approximately 1 cm mesial and distal to the site is adequate.
2. A full-thickness envelope flap is then elevated. Vertical releasing incisions may be necessary for exposure; however, this may lead to a greater amount of patient discomfort postoperatively. Extensive flap reflection may lead to devitalization of bone and should be avoided.

3. The degree of bony abnormality will dictate the most effective method for alveoloplasty. Smaller irregularities at an extraction site may only require digital compression of the socket walls. A rongeur, bone file, handpiece with bur, or a mallet and osteotome are all viable options for bony recontouring (**Fig. 1**). Irrigation with normal saline during the procedure is critical to maintain bony temperature less than 47°C.[6]

4. The site is inspected carefully and irrigated copiously with normal saline. Undetected residual free bony fragments may lead to delayed postoperative healing or possibly infection.

5. The mucoperiosteal flap is reapproximated and the site palpated to ensure removal of all irregularities. Excess soft tissue should also be removed at this time. The flap is then closed with a running resorbable suture, as fewer knots may be more comfortable and hygienic for patients.[7]

Historically, intraseptal alveoloplasty offers an alternative technique to remove large bony undercuts while maintaining vertical ridge height (**Fig. 2**). However, this method should be used judiciously while maintaining adequate ridge width to accommodate possible future implant placement.[7]

Maxillary Tuberosity Reduction

The intermaxillary space necessary for proper prosthesis fabrication may be decreased because of vertical excess of the maxillary tuberosity. Generally, the intermaxillary distance should be at least 1 cm when patients are placed into the correct or planned vertical dimension of occlusion.[4] A dental mirror passing freely between the tuberosity and retromolar tissue suggests adequate vertical clearance. The mirror can then be placed on the lateral aspect of the tuberosity, and patients are instructed to open and close. If the mirror intrudes on the mandible's path during function, horizontal reduction of the tuberosity may be required. A determination as to the extent of soft tissue and bony contribution to the problem is made radiographically. A panoramic view is recommended to ensure an adequate assessment of the relationship between the maxillary sinus and residual alveolus, particularly if bony reduction is contemplated.

1. Local anesthetic with epinephrine is administered, and a crestal linear or elliptical incision is made from the posterior tuberosity to a point anterior to the site of interest (**Fig. 3**). When an

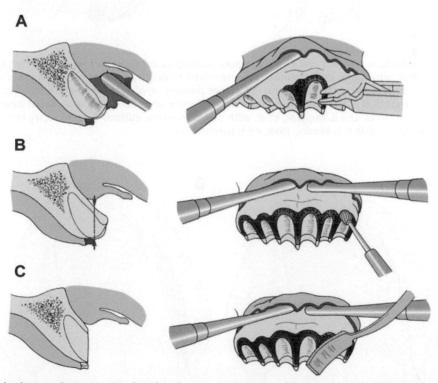

Fig. 1. Alveoloplasty techniques using hand and rotary instruments. (*A*) Flap elevation, alveoloplasty using rongeurs. (*B*) Alveoloplasty using rotary instrumentation. (*C*) Final contouring and smoothing using a bone file. (*From* Peterson LJ, Ellis E, Hupp JR, et al, with six contributors, editors. Contemporary oral and maxillofacial surgery. St Louis (MO): C.V. Mosby; 1988; with permission.)

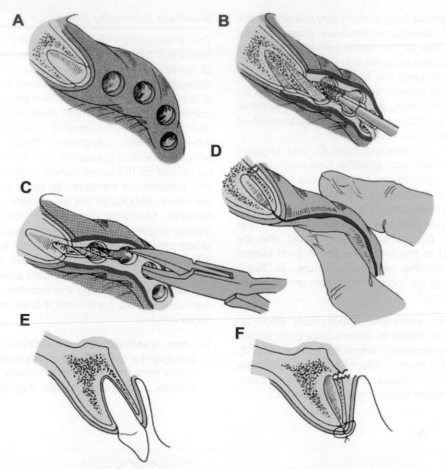

Fig. 2. Intraseptal bone is removed and digital pressure applied to collapse ridge and eliminate undercuts. (*A*) Alveolar bone after extractions. (*B*) Intraseptal bone removed to depth of socket with rotary instrumentation. (*C*) Intraseptal bone removed with a rongeur. (*D*) Finger pressure applied to in-fracture labial plate of bone and eliminate undercuts. (*E*) Cross-sectional view of pre-extraction alveolus. (*F*) Cross-sectional view after alveoloplasty. (*From* Peterson LJ, Ellis E, Hupp JR, et al, with six contributors, editors. Contemporary oral and maxillofacial surgery. St Louis (MO): C.V. Mosby; 1988; with permission.)

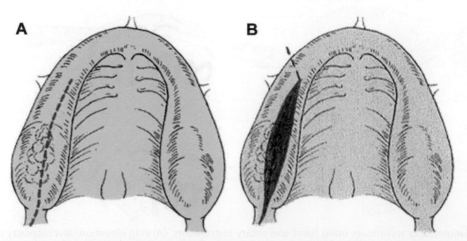

Fig. 3. Incisions for tuberosity reduction: (*A*) Single crestal incision (*red dashed line*) used when minimal reduction is planned. (*B*) Elliptical incision with anterior release. (*From* Peterson LJ, Ellis E, Hupp JR, et al, with six contributors, editors. Contemporary oral and maxillofacial surgery. St Louis (MO): C.V. Mosby; 1988; with permission.)

elliptical design is selected, the width of the ellipse is estimated by the magnitude of anticipated tissue removal. The buccal side of the ellipse is placed first, well within the zone of attached tissue. When minimal reduction is anticipated, a single crestal incision may be used.

2. Before flap elevation, excess fibrous tissue is removed by undermining the mucosa with a beveled incision and excising a wedge on the palatal side of the wound and, if indicated, on the buccal side as well (**Fig. 4**A).

3. A buccal release at the anterior end of the incision provides significantly enhanced access and visibility, particularly when horizontal as well as vertical bony reduction is planned. The mucoperiosteal flap is then elevated in both buccal and palatal directions allowing access to the bony tuberosity (see **Fig. 4**B).

4. Depending on the circumstances and operator preference, bone can be removed with hand and/or rotary instruments (see **Fig. 4**C). The site should be smoothed with a bone file, inspected for residual bony fragments, and irrigated copiously with normal saline.

5. Any excess soft tissue can be excised from the palatal aspect as this side of the wound has unlimited keratinized, attached tissue. The site is then closed with a running resorbable suture (see **Fig. 4**D).

In the case of solely soft tissue tuberosity reduction, excess tissue can be removed by simple wedge resection. Tension free closure is then achieved by undermining the buccal and palatal flaps subperiosteally. Additional submucosal tissue can be undermined and removed to aid in closure (**Fig. 5**).

Torus Removal

The cause of maxillary and mandibular tori is unclear.[8] In dentate individuals, removal is often unnecessary unless normal speech, mastication, or general patient comfort is affected. However, after teeth are lost, tori may complicate or even preclude denture fabrication. Large, lobulated tori with undercuts must be treated, whereas the restoring dentist may deem smaller, smooth, broad-based tori insignificant.

Maxillary (palatal) torus removal

Before surgery, potential complications should be discussed with patients, including wound dehiscence, prolonged pain, and oral-nasal

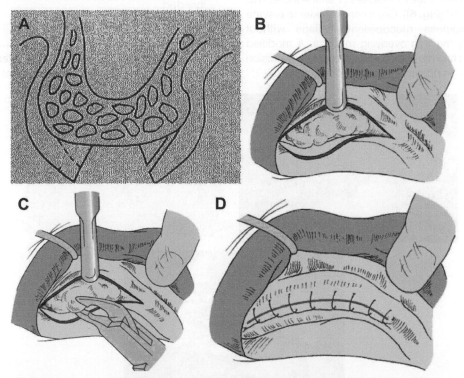

Fig. 4. (*A*) Beveled incision to eliminate bulky tissue while preserving mucosa. (*B*) Elevation of buccal and palatal mucoperiosteal flaps. (*C*) Removal of excess bone from the tuberosity. (*D*) Closure with interlocking continuous suture technique. (*Courtesy of* [*A*] Alan Samit, DDS, West Orange, NJ; and *From* [*B*, *C*] Peterson LJ, Ellis E, Hupp JR, et al, with six contributors, editors. Contemporary oral and maxillofacial surgery. St Louis (MO): C.V. Mosby; 1988; with permission.)

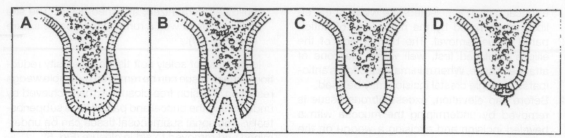

Fig. 5. Soft tissue tuberosity reduction. (*A*) Maxillary tuberosity with excess soft tissue. (*B*) Removal of tissue between buccal and palatal arms of the incision. (*C*) Flap edges after undermining and removing excess tissue. (*D*) Primary closure after any necessary mucosal trimming. (*From* Fonseca RJ, Davis WH. Reconstructive preprosthetic oral and maxillofacial surgery. St Louis (MO): W.B. Saunders; 1986; with permission.)

communication caused by thin overlying palatal bone following torus removal. A maxillary impression is taken and study model poured. The torus is then removed from the cast until flush with the surrounding palate, and a splint is formed with relief provided in the area of the torus. The splint may be made from acrylic or thermoplastic (suck down) material. Soft tissue liner may be used when the splint is placed postoperatively to aid in patient comfort and prevent hematoma formation.

1. Local anesthesia with epinephrine is administered, and a midline incision is made with posterior and/or anterior releases (Y shape incision at each end [**Fig. 6**]). Great care is taken to elevate full-thickness mucoperiosteal flaps without tearing the thin overlying mucosa. A modified palatal flap has been described to avoid incision lines over possible palatal perforations.[9]

2. Depending on the size of the torus and the nature of its attachment to the underlying bone, removal may be accomplished with rongeurs, a rotary instrument with an acrylic bur, or a mallet and osteotome. It is recommended that large tori be sectioned with a fissure bur and then removed with the mallet and osteotome. Final contouring is done with an egg-shaped bur and/or bone file.

3. The site is irrigated copiously with normal saline. Excess soft tissue may be trimmed, and the flaps are reapproximated with interrupted resorbable sutures.

4. The stent is relined with tissue conditioner and inserted.

Removal of Mandibular Tori

1. Local anesthesia is achieved with inferior alveolar and lingual blocks. Infiltration at the site

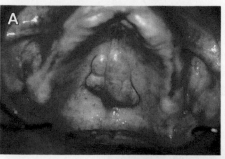

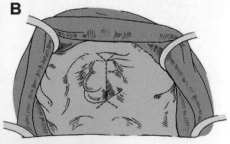

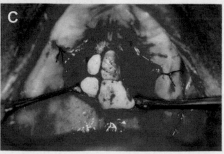

Fig. 6. Palatal torus removal. (*A*) Palatal torus. (*B*) Incision design. (*C*) Exposure of the palatal torus with retraction sutures. (*From* Peterson LJ, Ellis E, Hupp JR, et al, with six contributors, editors. Contemporary oral and maxillofacial surgery. St Louis (MO): C.V. Mosby; 1988; with permission.)

may aid in hemostasis as well as facilitate dissection.

2. Incision over the crest of the ridge, or along the lingual sulcus of teeth when present, is made with extension to ensure adequate visualization of the tori to be removed. Vertical incisions may interfere with the blood supply to the thin overlying mucosa covering the tori and should be avoided[4] (**Fig. 7**).

3. Elevation of the delicate lingual mucoperiosteal flap requires great care. A periosteal elevator or Seldin retractor is placed beneath the torus to protect the floor of the mouth during removal.

4. Depending on the size of the torus and the nature of its attachment to the underlying bone, removal may be accomplished with rongeurs, a rotary instrument with an acrylic bur, or a mallet and osteotome. A trough to guide proper osteotome cleavage can be created initially with a bur paralleling the lingual cortex to avoid unfavorable fractures. Final contouring is done with an egg-shaped bur or bone file. Specially designed bur guards are available that help protect the lingual soft tissues by exposing only the surface of the bur in contact with the bone (**Fig. 8**). S-shaped bone files are designed for smoothing on the lingual surface of the mandible and their use is recommended.

5. The site is irrigated copiously with normal saline; the tissue is adapted and palpated for irregularities, and closure is achieved with a running resorbable suture.

6. Some sources advise placement of a gauze pack under the tongue in the floor of the mouth for approximately 6 to 12 hours to prevent hematoma formation.[6]

SOFT TISSUE PROCEDURES
Frenectomy

Many maxillary dentures are fabricated working around a pronounced labial frenum (**Fig. 9**A). The result is a deeply notched prosthesis, irritation of the mucosa, and the loss of surface area that might otherwise contribute to retention and stability. A variety of frenectomy techniques are used; but if the moveable tissue interposed between mucosa and periosteum is not addressed, the frenectomy is incomplete as a preprosthetic procedure.

The maxillary labial frenectomy for denture patients should be a limited submucosal

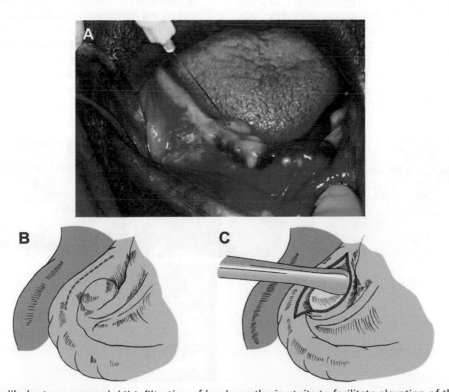

Fig. 7. Mandibular torus removal. (*A*) Infiltration of local anesthesia at site to facilitate elevation of thin mucosa overlying a mandibular torus. (*B*) Incision placed over the alveolar crest. (*C*) Flap elevation to ensure adequate access and allow retractor placement to protect the floor of the mouth. (*From* Peterson LJ, Ellis E, Hupp JR, et al, with six contributors, editors. Contemporary oral and maxillofacial surgery. St Louis (MO): C.V. Mosby; 1988; with permission.)

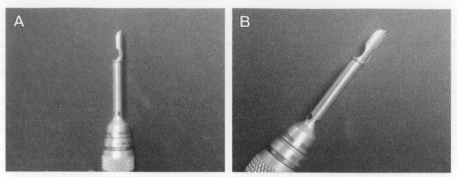

Fig. 8. (*A*, *B*) Bur guard designed to protect lingual tissues during mandibular torus removal.

vestibuloplasty. Instrumentation is minimal: a pair of Dean (or similar) scissors, a needle holder, and a local anesthetic syringe. One specific requirement is a 3-0 or 4-0 suture on a taper needle.

1. After local anesthesia administration, the lip is retracted upward and the frenal connection to the alveolus is cut with the scissors continuing superiorly until a diamond-shaped wound is created (see **Fig. 9**B).
2. The scissors are then held parallel to the alveolar bone and used to perform submucosal and supraperiosteal dissections for 1 to 2 cm on both sides of the wound (see **Fig. 9**C). This procedure produces 2 tunnels: one submucosal and the other supraperiosteal (see **Fig. 9**D).
3. The scissors are then turned so that the cutting surfaces are perpendicular to the alveolar bone and used to cut the moveable tissue between the submucosal and supraperiosteal tunnels. The cut is made as inferiorly as possible so that all of the submucosal tissue can retract upward. The scissors may be used to push the tissue superiorly so that only mucosa and periosteum remain in the denture-bearing area.
4. The height of the vestibule is then established by passing a suture through one mucosal edge, engaging periosteum, coming through the mucosal edge on the opposite side of the wound, and tying the suture to tack the mucosa to periosteum. The use of a taper needle is critical as the periosteum is delicate, tightly bound to bone, and may be torn if a cutting needle is used. At least one additional pass above and below the initial suture is generally indicated. Periosteum may be engaged again where possible, but this is critical only with the first tacking suture (see **Fig. 9**E).

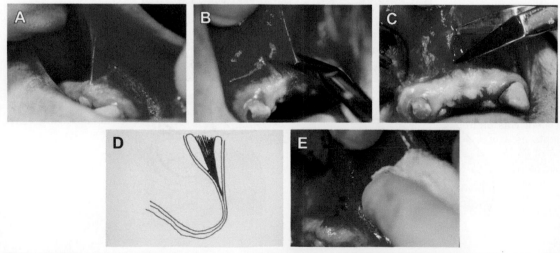

Fig. 9. (*A*) Hyperplastic maxillary labial frenum. (*B*) Incision at base of frenum with Dean scissors. (*C*) Submucosal and supraperiosteal dissection. (*D*) Cross-sectional view of submucosal and supraperiosteal tunnels. (*E*) Completed frenectomy with the new vestibular height established by periosteal tacking suture. (*Courtesy of* [*D*] Alan Samit, DDS, West Orange, NJ.)

Submucosal vestibuloplasty techniques have been used to address entire maxillary arches with the dissections described earlier carried as far as possible from the midline incision. When treating an entire arch, a stent has been used to maintain vestibular integrity.[4]

Submucosal vestibuloplasty techniques create a zone of immobile denture-bearing tissue, but they do not change the quality of the tissue. Use of the submucosal vestibuloplasty in the mandible puts the mental nerves at risk, and Obwegeser[5] recommended that the procedure be limited to the maxilla.[4]

Skin Grafting

The concept of transplanting skin to cover open wounds has a long history. A definitive article on the Thiersch graft published in 1934 by T.P. Kilner,[10] a London plastic surgeon, describes indications, techniques, and care of patients. Although some of this has changed over the last 80 years, much of Kilner's work is still relevant. Free skin grafts survive over the first few days by imbibition and then inosculation as vascular connections are established. This phase is followed by neovascularization and the development of a firm connection between the graft and recipient bed. Ultimately, a well-healed intraoral skin graft becomes part of the denture-bearing area with positive characteristics, including immobility, favorable texture, and a good response to load bearing and irritation.

Vestibuloplasty

The skin graft vestibuloplasty with lowering of the floor of the mouth offers several advantages over other methods of preparing the edentulous mandible for a complete denture. With good patient selection and surgical technique, this procedure can transform a moderately atrophic mandible with unfavorable soft tissue attachments into an excellent bed for a comfortable and functional prosthesis. The traditional procedure using a stent was unpopular among surgeons and patients as it was a long, laborious operation with an often unpleasant postoperative course. Complications related to the stent, the awl passes, graft take, and donor site morbidity, made the procedure unattractive despite its ability to produce dramatic changes.[11] Modifications were proposed, and the procedure evolved into a more reasonable option for patients and surgeons.[12] The modified version described later eliminates the need for a stent, reduces the number of awl passes, cuts operating time to less than 2 hours, and is associated with a relatively benign postoperative course

with minimal morbidity. Clearly, an implant-borne prosthesis is superior to one that rests on the tissues. Nonetheless, the skin graft vestibuloplasty is a versatile procedure that is potentially transformative for patients who are not candidates for implants and may be beneficial for those who have implant-supported but partially tissue-borne prostheses.

The procedure as described by Samit and Popowich[13] is based on a careful review of several cases done using the traditional method. The modified procedure is highly predictable and successful with few significant complications.[14,15]

The stent was a frequent source of inaccuracy and required additional awl passes. Grafts inadequately adapted to the recipient bed were lost as were those under excessive pressure from the stent. It was noted that graft failure labially invariably led to significant loss of vestibular depth, whereas the lingual vestibular extension was stable regardless of the status of the graft.

Modifications
Eliminate the stent and place the skin graft on the labial only suturing it directly to periosteum with a taper needle. The number of awl passes Is reduced to 4:2 anterior and 2 posterior to the mental nerves.

Hematoma under the graft is possible even when it is sewn directly to periosteum.

Modification
Using an 18-gauge needle or No. 11 blade, the graft is fenestrated at the end of the procedure taking care not to cut sutures or injure the mental nerves.

Floor-of-mouth swelling has been reported and, in some case, interfered with salivary flow. Dexamethasone injection into the floor of the mouth and cannulation of the submandibular ducts were advocated. Prophylactic antibiotics were used to cover the awl passes.

Modifications
Intravenous dexamethasone is effective without the risks associated with injection into the floor of the mouth. With fewer awl passes and careful management of floor-of-mouth tissues, prophylactic cannulation of the submandibular ducts is not necessary. There is no evidence to support the use of prophylactic antibiotics. Localized abscesses at the site of awl passes on skin are rare and may be managed with incision, drainage, and antibiotics, if indicated.

The donor site was expansive and a source of significant pain in the postoperative period.

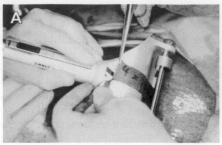
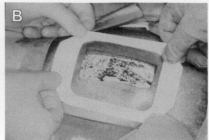

Fig. 10. (*A*) Split-thickness skin graft harvest using a dermatome. (*B*) Placement of a semiporous membrane over the donor site.

Modifications

A skin graft capable of successfully treating an entire labial vestibule can be derived from a donor site as small as 2 by 5 cm. A semiporous adhesive membrane (Opsite [Smith+Nephew, London, UK], Tegaderm [3M Corp., St. Paul, MN]) is used to dress the donor site, and patients report minimal or no pain and can bathe and dress normally.

Extensive and highly detailed descriptions of the traditional procedure appear in the literature.[4] Many of the elements of the modified, stentless technique are similar, with major modifications noted earlier. The steps involved are presented in outline form:

1. Graft harvest using a dermatome is most often from a hairless area on the upper lateral thigh. Antibacterial skin preparations are made followed by alcohol to remove all stickiness from the surface. A liberal application of mineral oil to the skin and the dermatome provides needed lubrication.
2. A marked site measuring between 2.0 and 2.5 by 5 to 6 cm is harvested and set epithelial side up on a hard surface, such as the bottom of a kidney basin, and covered with a saline sponge. If the skin is not marked before harvest, note the direction it curls: always inward toward the dermal side (**Fig. 10**).
3. The labial dissection begins with a molar-to-molar mucosal incision at the mucogingival

junction, which is generally near the crest on these cases. Using a tissue scissors with a snip-and-push technique, the mucosa and all loose, moveable supraperiosteal tissues are moved inferiorly (**Fig. 11**).
4. La Grange scissors or similar instrument is used to remove all remnants of moveable tissue remaining on the periosteum as these are gently pulled away from the periosteal bed using a Frazier-tip surgical suction.
5. The lingual incision should be slightly shorter in length than the labial; the blade is held parallel to the alveolus, not facing the bone. A sponge stick is used to tense the floor of the mouth so that the incision can be made as described earlier without jeopardizing the delicate lingual periosteum (**Fig. 12**).
6. Dissection on the lingual is easily accomplished with a gloved finger. Four lengths of a 2-0 chromic suture are attached to the cut lingual mucosal edge: 2 on each side of the midline, one placed posteriorly, and the other more anterior. The needles are removed and the 4 sutures are held in order on snaps in preparation for awl passes (**Fig. 13**).
7. Using a standard technique, 4 submandibular passes are made with an awl after skin prep and puncture with a No. 11 blade. At each site, the ends of each of the 4 sutures are picked up lingually and brought around to the facial side where one end is removed

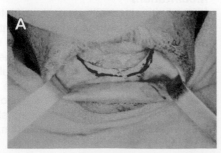
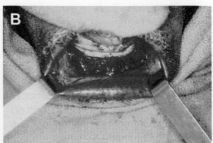

Fig. 11. (*A*) Labial incision: note preservation of crestal attached gingiva. (*B*) Labial dissection: note development of extensive periosteal bed free of moveable tissue.

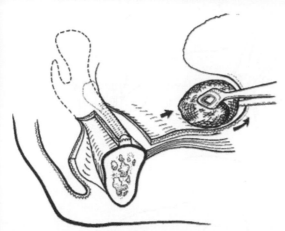

Fig. 12. Use of a sponge stick for traction to facilitate the lingual incision. (*From* Fonseca RJ, Davis WH. Reconstructive preprosthetic oral and maxillofacial surgery. St Louis (MO): W.B. Saunders; 1986; with permission.)

from the eye of the awl at the base of the vestibule and the other is passed through the cut edge of the mucosa. The 4 sutures are tied in succession with the assistant's gloved finger in the lingual vestibule ensuring that the mucosal edge is secured inferiorly (**Fig. 14**).

8. The labial mucosal edge will require additional attachment to periosteum. This attachment is accomplished with a 3-0 chromic suture on a taper needle. The mucosa should be sutured to the periosteum as low in the vestibule as possible tacking the loose edges between and behind the awl-passed suture ties.

9. Should this require a tacking suture near the mental nerve, the taper needle should be passed through the mucosal edge, then engage the periosteum under the nerve with the needle traveling posterior to anterior. Instead of tying the ends at this point, which would damage the nerve, the needle is passed back through periosteum under the nerve from anterior to posterior and back through the mucosa in mattress fashion. Using this technique, the mucosa is tightly bound to the periosteum without constructing the nerve.

10. The skin is divided into two by making a semi-diagonal cut through the rectangular graft (**Fig. 15**). With the surgical suction eliminated from the field to preclude inadvertent loss of the skin graft, a 3-0 chromic suture on a cutting needle is used to attach one of the sections of skin to one side of the recipient bed. The suture is passed through the corner of the skin graft and attached to residual tissue just superior to the edge of the recipient bed in a continuous fashion while stretching the skin posteriorly with each suture pass. This procedure is repeated on the opposite side so that the site is covered with skin widest at the midline, with the dermal side of the graft facing the periosteum.

11. The process is completed by tacking the two skin sections together at the midline using a 3-0 chromic on a taper needle. The inferior edge is also tacked to the periosteum (not to the mucosa) using the same material and technique with the skin stretched gently so that it lies flat on the periosteal bed. Excess skin may be trimmed as needed.

12. Finally, a No. 11 blade or needle is used to fenestrate the graft. Multiple small punctures are made through the skin down to bone, carefully avoiding sutures and the mental nerves. This, along with a pressure bandage placed across the chin, makes hematoma

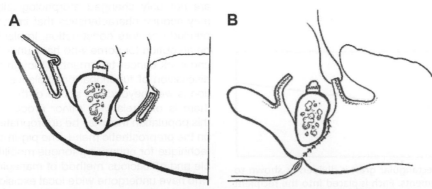

Fig. 13. (*A*) Lingual dissection accomplished by the gentle use of a gloved finger. (*B*) Suture placed through the mucosal edge of the lingual flap. The awl will be introduced through a submandibular cutaneous puncture.

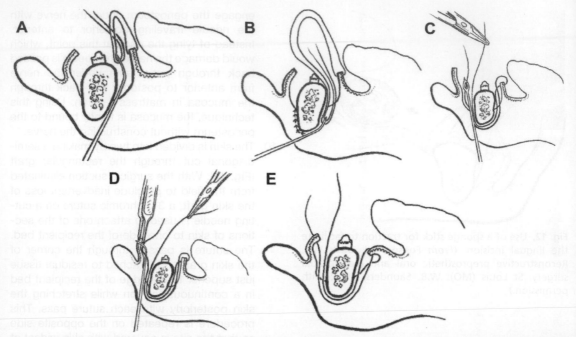

Fig. 14. (*A*) Both ends of the suture are fed through the eye of the awl. (*B*) The awl is withdrawn and carefully brought around the inferior border of the mandible without exiting the skin. (*C*) The awl is passed into the labio-buccal vestibule. This technique is done for each of the 4 sutures, right and left, anterior and posterior to the mental nerve. (*D*) One end of the suture is removed from the eye of the awl, and the awl is then passed through the mucosa near the edge of the labio-buccal flap. (*E*) The suture is now ready to be tied down lowering the floor of the mouth and securing the labio-buccal mucosa at its new vestibular depth. (*From* [*E*] Fonseca RJ, Davis WH. Reconstructive preprosthetic oral and maxillofacial surgery. St Louis (MO): W.B. Saunders; 1986; with permission.)

formation unlikely and allows the graft to remain well adapted during the critical early stages of healing.

Donor site management and oral wound care are performed as have been described for any type of skin graft. The most critical instruction to patients is to ensure that no alcohol comes into contact with the graft for the first 10 to 14 days. Mouthwashes as well as alcoholic beverages will interfere with graft healing.

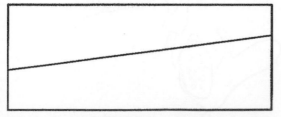

Fig. 15. The rectangular graft is divided as shown to produce 2 segments. Each is placed into the recipient bed, tacking the wider end at the midline and working posteriorly, right and left.

Sloughing of outer layers of the graft is expected at week one; but by week 4 the graft is well adapted, and impressions may be taken by the restoring dentist to begin the restorative phase of treatment (**Fig. 16**).

Other Skin Graft Procedures

Prosthodontic rehabilitation of patients with oral cancer is a major challenge. Denture-bearing tissues affected by surgery and/or radiation therapy are not only changed morphologically but also may acquire characteristics that impede or even preclude denture construction. Implants may not be an option for some who have undergone head and neck cancer treatment. Although a complete discussion of functional postablative reconstruction is well beyond the scope of this publication, there is one relatively minor procedure used in this population that may be appropriately included on the preprosthetic menu. The pig-in-the-blanket technique for enhancing tongue mobility is a simple and efficacious method of managing patients who have undergone wide local excision of lateral tongue/floor-of-the-mouth squamous cell carcinoma. In these patients, there is often scarring

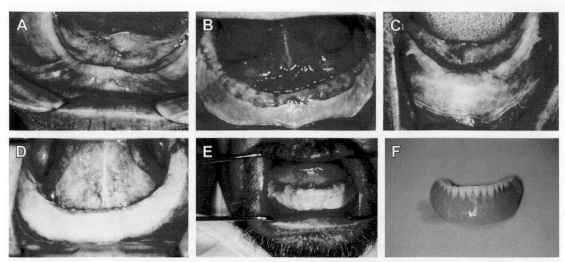

Fig. 16. (*A*) Preoperative view demonstrating shallow vestibules with superiorly positioned muscle attachments and a minimal zone of crestal attached tissue. (*B*) Postoperative view with well-adapted skin graft, significant labio-buccal vestibular depth, and floor of mouth lowered. (*C*) Postoperative view with well-adapted skin graft: note skin pigmentation maintained at the recipient site. (*D*) Postoperative view with well-adapted skin graft, significant labio-buccal vestibular depth, and floor of mouth lowered. (*E*) Postoperative view with well-adapted skin graft, significant labio-buccal vestibular depth, and floor of mouth lowered. (*F*) Prosthesis demonstrating maximal extension fabricated after skin graft vestibuloplasty.

that binds the tongue laterally and obliterates the lingual vestibule. This scarring limits tongue mobility and makes it very difficult, if not impossible, to fabricate a functional prosthesis. Skin grafting may be considered 1 year after treatment of the cancer provided there is no evidence of recurrence or a new primary at that time.

1. An incision is made into the scarred area where a lingual vestibule would normally be. This incision is carried to a depth that provides separation and some degree of freedom for the tongue while respecting local anatomy.
2. Skin will have been harvested as described earlier with the graft size estimated by the anticipated surface area of the defect. The skin is attached to the periphery of the defect and stretched gently as it is sutured so that the defect is lined with skin that is taut and well adapted.
3. Additional resorbable sutures may be used to tack the skin to the muscle bed, and a No. 11 blade or needle may be used to fenestrate the graft to reduce the likelihood of hematoma formation.
4. A roll of saline-moistened sterile gauze is placed in the defect, and the original incision line is closed with silk. The gauze puts gentle pressure on the skin, which then adapts well to both sides of the defect (**Fig. 17**).
5. The silk sutures are removed along with the gauze roll in 7 to 10 days. A vestibular fold is

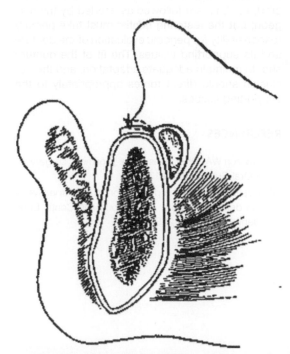

Fig. 17. The wound is closed to the original incision line after suturing in the skin graft and inserting a roll of saline-moistened gauze to maintain pressure against the recipient bed. (*From* Leban SG. The use of a modified skin grafting technique for alveolar sulcus extension. J Oral Surg 1977;35:553; with permission.)

produced that is lined by skin, and there is generally a significant improvement in tongue mobility.

Care must be taken to ensure that graft healing continues with appropriate instructions given to patients and dietary restrictions imposed for an additional 1 to 2 weeks.

SUMMARY

The delivery of a prosthesis that meets the Lawson criteria often requires collaboration between the surgeon and the restoring dentist. Preprosthetic surgery should always be considered for patients receiving conventional dentures as well as for those who will have prostheses that are partially implant borne.[16] Preoperatively this involves a careful and critical evaluation of the relevant anatomy and a shared vision of what is necessary to optimize the function and esthetics of the planned prosthesis. Intraoperatively, each procedure should be carried out with the intent of maximizing the contours, quantity, and quality of denture-bearing tissues. Postoperatively, the surgeon ensures that healing is adequate before prosthesis fabrication begins. Once the prosthesis is delivered, patients are followed as needed by the surgeon; but the restoring dentist must take primary responsibility for periodic evaluation of the denture and its supporting tissues. The fit of the denture should maintain adequate adaptation, and the occlusion should direct forces appropriately to the supporting tissues.

REFERENCES

1. Lawson WA. Objectives of pre-prosthetic surgery. Br J Oral Surg 1972;10:175–88.
2. Castelberry DJ. The prosthodontist's perspective of the deficient alveolar ridge. Compend Contin Educ Dent 1982;(suppl 2):S49–51.
3. Peterson LJ, Ellis E, Hupp JR, Tucker MR, With six contributors, editors. Contemporary oral and maxillofacial surgery. St Louis (MO): C. V. Mosby; 1988.
4. Fonseca RJ, Davis WH. Reconstructive preprosthetic oral and maxillofacial surgery. St Louis (MO): W. B. Saunders; 1986.
5. Obwegeser H. Die submukose vestibulumplastik. Dtsch Zahnarztl Z 1959;14:629, 749.
6. Eriksson RA, Albrektsson T. Temperature threshold levels for heat-induced bone tissue injury. A vital microscopic study in the rabbit. J Prosthet Dent 1983;50:101.
7. Miloro M, Ghali GE, Larson PE, et al, editors. Waite: Peterson's principles of oral and maxillofacial surgery. 3rd edition. Shelton, CT: PMPH USA; 2011.
8. García-García AS, Martínez-González JM, Gómez-Font R, et al. Current status of the torus palatinus and torus mandibularis. Med Oral Patol Oral Cir Bucal 2010;15:E353.
9. Chacko JP, Joseph C. Modified palatal flap: a simpler approach for removal of palatal tori. J Oral Maxillofac Surg 2010;68(4):943–4.
10. Kilner TP. The Thiersch graft: its preparation and uses. Postgrad Med J 1934;10:176–81.
11. Steinhauser EW. Vestibuloplasty – skin grafts. J Oral Surg 1971;29:777–85.
12. Leban SG. The use of a modified skin grafting technique for alveolar sulcus extension. J Oral Surg 1977;35:552–4.
13. Samit A, Popowich L. Mandibular vestibuloplasty: a clinical update. Oral Surg Oral Med Oral Pathol 1982;54:141–7.
14. Popowich L, Samit A. Respiratory obstruction following vestibuloplasty and lowering of the floor of the mouth. J Oral Maxillofac Surg 1983;41:255–7.
15. Samit A, Kent K. Complications associated with skin graft vestibuloplasty – experiences with 100 cases. Oral Surg Oral Med Oral Pathol 1983;56:586–92.
16. Cillo JE Jr, Finn R. Reconstruction of the shallow vestibule edentulous mandible with simultaneous split thickness skin graft vestibuloplasty and mandibular endosseous implants for implant-supported overdentures. J Oral Maxillofac Surg 2009;67:381–6.

Index

Note: Page numbers of article titles are in **boldface** type.

Oral Maxillofacial Surg Clin N Am 27 (2015) 473–478

http://dx.doi.org/10.1016/S1042-3699(15)00065-5

1042-3699/15/$ – see front matter © 2015 Elsevier Inc. All rights reserved.

oralmaxsurgery.theclinics.com

Printed and bound by CPI Group (UK) Ltd, Croydon, CR0 4YY

03/10/2024

01040374-0006